THE NEW GRAD

How To Become A Competent, Confident and Competitive New Grad Physio

Andy Barker

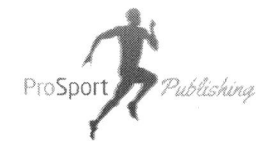

ProSport *Publishing*

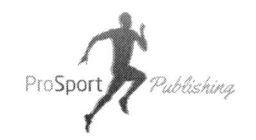

ISBN: 978-1-091-02808-1

Copyright © 2019 Andy Barker

A CIP record for this book is available from the British Library

The moral right of the author has been asserted

All rights reserved

The Copyright Act prohibits (subject to certain very limited exceptions) the making of copies of any copyright work or of a substantial part of such a work, including the making of copies by photocopying or similar process. Written permission to make a copy or copies must therefore normally be obtained from the publisher in advance. It is advisable also to consult the publisher if in any doubt as to the legality of any copying which is to be undertaken.

Edited and typeset by Helen Jones

Facebook @NewGradPhysio
Instagram @NewGradPhysio

Dedication

I firstly would like to thank my parents for the support they have given me over the years particularly in helping me through my education. This support has enabled me to follow my career dreams; without it my road to this point might have been very different.

So many others have guided my own development as a therapist. I am indebted to the help given to me by David O'Sullivan as he helped me through those early years, giving me the clinical and non-clinical skills needed to accelerate my own career as a New Grad Physio.

The biggest thank you must go to my wife Sammy. She's been there right from the start of my own New Grad journey after we first met at university. She's been there supporting me every step of the way; as well as supporting me, she is a fantastic mother to our two boys, Blake and Kit.

Lastly, I would like to thank the hundreds of New Grad Physios I have worked with and coached, especially those currently part of the New Grad Physio Membership. These therapists have helped guide the content for this book and without them this publication would not have been possible.

CONTENTS

Foreword vi

What everyone else is saying about Andy Barker
and The New Grad Physio Membership viii

CHAPTER 1 The struggles of a New Grad Physio 13

CHAPTER 2 My story – new grad to 'dream job' in just 15 months 20

CHAPTER 3 The biggest misconceptions and mistakes
ALL new grads make.. 32

CHAPTER 4 The New Grad Physio way... 43

CHAPTER 5 **Competency 1** How to get noticed and gain entry
to your first role in the NHS, private practice or sport 53

CHAPTER 6 **Competency 2** How to SURVIVE as a New Grad Physio.... 72

CHAPTER 7 **Competency 3** How to not only survive but THRIVE
as a New Grad Physio 86

CHAPTER 8 **Competency 4** How to get your next promotion 105

CHAPTER 9 How to hit the ground running in the NHS
as a New Grad Physio 130

CHAPTER 10 How to overcome the challenges
of a New Grad Physio working in private practice 141

CHAPTER 11 How to excel working in professional sport as a New Grad Physio 150

CHAPTER 12 A day in the life of a New Grad Physio 161

CHAPTER 13 The fastest way to becoming a competent, confident and successful New Grad Physio and progressing up the promotion ladder 175

CHAPTER 14 New Grad Physio members in focus 188

About The New Grad Physio Mentor, Andy Barker 191

New Grad Physio Bonus Resources 192

Foreword

Welcome to *The New Grad Physio*!

The New Grad Physio was born out of my own frustrations and challenges as a New Grad Physio and the subsequent similar issues other New Grad therapists struggle with day after day. Receiving question after question from frustrated New Grad Physios was becoming a daily occurrence.

Like me, New Grads transitioning out of university and into employment were finding it difficult to navigate the early challenges that all New Grad therapists face.

During my own studies some therapists gave up. They couldn't cope with the demands put on them by the fast-paced, intense therapy degree. Additionally, some therapists did qualify, but within those early years gave up on the therapy profession and pursued something else.

This is one end of the spectrum but so many therapists I have previously worked with tell me stories about their loss of motivation, drive and passion for the profession. In short, they have stopped enjoying the job they always wanted to do.

I'm sure you've already experienced how rewarding and fulfilling life as a therapist can be when you are able to make changes to patients' pain and get them back to function.

However, on the flip side, when you struggle to make changes clinically, when your patients don't get better, and when you can't quite grasp what is going on, it can be very lonely and frustrating. You are left feeling that you are doing your patients a disservice by not giving them the high-quality care they deserve.

Upon completion of our studies, we are qualified, we are expected to know everything, and our patients expect results. But no New Grad Physio is the finished article straight out of university. I know from my own journey how difficult those first years are as a New Grad and how much help and support you will need if you are to overcome the challenges that you face.

Maybe you've not quite qualified but have heard how scarily different life as a New Grad Physio can be: very different to what we were led to believe by our university lecturers.

If you haven't heard this already, then IT IS VERY DIFFERENT!

I also know from personal experience and from my work coaching other New Grad Physios that the main difference between those New Grads that are successful and those that are not, is the access to help and support. And that is exactly why I put together the New Grad Physio Membership.

I want to help as many New Grad Physios as I can to overcome the barriers and challenges and to become better therapists. I want other New Grads to be able to achieve their dream job, just like I was able to do, to be able to help their patients out of pain and back to function and, most importantly, start enjoying their jobs.

This book will guide you through the main challenges you will face; these are the same challenges you MUST overcome if you are to become a competent, confident and competitive New Grad Physio.

To find out more about the New Grad Physio Membership visit
www.newgradphysio.com

Here's to your successful New Grad journey...

Andy Barker **MSc BSc MCSP**

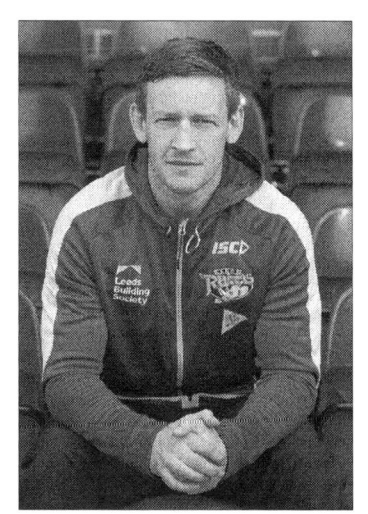

What everyone else is saying about Andy Barker and The New Grad Physio Membership

David O'Sullivan, Head Physiotherapist England Rugby League
'I made a lot of mistakes starting out initially as a New Grad; it was really a process of trial and error. I was lucky to have a great mentor who helped me avoid some BIG mistakes with BIGGER consequences… From here it took me a few years to make sense of WHY things were happening which is why what Andy is doing, helping New Grads gain confidence & clarity and get accurate results with their patient assessments, is greatly needed and a great investment as it will save you years of trying to figure it out yourself.'

Katie Davis, Chartered Senior Physiotherapist NHS and Private Practice
'When I first graduated, I found myself struggling with the time constraints of the initial assessment. Having a guide like the *New Grad Physio* to refer back to whenever I could would have saved so much of my time, just by being confident in doing my hands-on treatments and fully understanding how the body works.'

Shane Mooney, Chartered Senior Head Physiotherapist Private Practice
'When I first left university and started treating patients and athletes in the real world, it was a real eye-opener. Although I knew (or at least I thought I knew) theoretically what I needed to do, I found myself getting frustrated when I'd massage something or I'd use an exercise and get rid of someone's pain, only for them to come back next week telling me the pain had returned. It took a lot of trial and error to gain the confidence and clarity of exactly what my patient or athlete needed and when to progress them. I couldn't have done this without my mentors and I really wish I had had the New Grad Physio community and educational resource when I first started out!'

Chris Black, Head Of Physical Performance Leeds Rhinos

'Having worked with Andy for a number of seasons in elite sport I can honestly consider him to be one of the best physios in the business. Not only has he got exceptional knowledge of the human body, he also has a great understanding of where it all fits in the bigger picture of being a professional athlete. He has a genuine interest and passion of gym and field-based performance which makes him great to work with. I would highly recommend anyone who wants to gain valuable insight into being a top therapist in an applied setting to get involved with Andy.'

Keith Thornhill, Senior First Team Physiotherapist Munster Rugby Union

'I was lucky enough to work under Andy at Leeds Rhinos in my first full-time job in professional sport. During this time, I saw first-hand the experience, knowledge and drive which Andy possesses and uses daily to ensure that he gets the best results for his athletes.

'Andy has a proven track record of rehabilitating complex traumatic sporting injuries. He has proven that he can safely return his athletes to play far quicker than standard time frames but, more importantly, they are able to not only meet the demands of the sport but exceed them.

'Andy understands that the role of the therapist is different within public practice, private practice and sporting environments. I know that his New Grad Physio programme will not only be invaluable in helping you understand the demands of a therapist working in these areas but will also give you a sound understanding of the core principles needed to get the best results for your patients from the outset of your career.'

Ben Harper, Private Practice Owner & Lead Physio British Taekwondo

'Andy has been a colleague, mentor and now close friend and clinic partner so I have first-hand experience of learning from his expertise. With bags of experience working at the top level of elite sport and private practice, he has the knowledge to give you the exposure and insight into the working mind and teach you the skill-sets needed to become a successful practitioner.

His New Grad Physio Membership will give an in-depth insight into the clinical decision-making and rationale of treatment approaches that a newly qualified clinician would only usually gain access to years into their career.'

Dr Jon Power, Consultant Sport & Exercise Medicine Doctor Football Association & Private Practice
'I've been fortunate enough to work with some excellent practitioners in the NHS, private clinics and elite sport. Andy Barker demonstrates the attributes needed to be a World Class practitioner daily. I'm certain he has the knowledge, skills, experience and credibility to help guide the next generation of therapists on their path towards a successful therapy career.'

Gareth Robinson, First Team Physiotherapist Leeds Rhinos
'I first met Andy after deciding on a career change and getting into full-time professional sport. Having been qualified for five years, I had experience working in a private practice, hospitals and part-time sport. I believed that I was well equipped to work in full-time sport but after a short period I realised just how much I still had to learn. Luckily Andy was the lead physiotherapist and my mentor; his knowledge, experience and guidance was invaluable. Although I know that I will never know everything in physiotherapy, Andy has provided me with a host of skills and knowledge that has given me confidence to provide a top-class physiotherapy service in any scenario. Andy is a brilliant physiotherapist and I recommend every New Grad therapist should join his New Grad Physio Membership – I certainly wish it had been available when I first qualified.'

Francesca Murphy, Sports Rehabilitator Private Practice & Professional Sport
'When I first graduated, I was overwhelmed by the 'real world' of sports medicine and injury. Without the guidance and advice given to me by Andy, I would not have got to where I am now. He has an invaluable wealth of knowledge on all elements of injury and the practical components of

gym-based rehabilitation. Andy's knowledge is based not only on thorough research, but also on its practical application, and he has shown me skill-sets that are tried and tested and work with real patients.

Andy sees the potential in New Grads across the disciplines; he knows how to mould them and guide them to become the best they can be. He shares his thoughts whilst taking your ideas on board, helping you to become autonomous and confident in assessing and treating an array of different patients and pathologies.'

James Wilkinson, Student MSc Physiotherapist & Sports Masseur

'As a current student physiotherapist, it has been vital to have Andy's advice and guidance to help me to develop my skills ready for graduation and the transition into working. Andy has helped me to reflect on my actions, building confidence in my own assessment and treatment skills. Having content like the *New Grad Physio* has been crucial to help me develop these skills, and the format of the membership allows me to access his advice and support whenever I like.'

To find out more about the New Grad Physio Membership or to contact Andy directly visit:

Website – www.newgradphysio.com

Email – andy@newgradphysio.com

Facebook - Search 'New Grad Physio Continuing Professional Development' or use this link:
https://www.facebook.com/newgradphysio

Instagram – Search 'new grad physio' or use this link:
https://www.instagram.com/newgradphysio

LinkedIn – Search 'Andy Barker' New Grad Physio or use this link:
https://uk.linkedin.com/in/andy-barker-b9118341

CHAPTER 1
The struggles of a New Grad Physio

The reality is that life as a New Grad Physio is tough.

No amount of university study and placement hours can prepare you for what is needed once you enter the REAL WORLD, working with REAL patients that expect REAL results.

Regardless of whether this is in the National Health Service (NHS), private practice or sport, the challenges remain the same. Many of the New Grad Physiotherapists, Sports Therapists and Sports Rehabilitators tell me the same stories, the same issues, the same challenges. If you are reading this book, it's likely you are encountering some of those challenges right now. Or if you are not, you soon will…

Despite the challenges being the same, why is it that some New Grads are seemingly able to quickly and easily overcome these challenges whilst others seem to get left behind?

Successful New Grad Physios get offered jobs straight away, maybe even before they've qualified. They can gain immediate respect and 'buy-in' from the patients they work with, meaning patients adhere to their treatment plans and as a result get better. They seem to thrive in their new surroundings and operate like experienced therapists; they can climb the career ladder quickly and get promoted to higher level roles.

On the flip side, some therapists really struggle. They struggle to get a job, sometimes even get an interview. Often this means they take a role they didn't really want, or a role they don't enjoy that leaves them feeling unsatisfied, undervalued and frustrated. In addition, they struggle to get patients to adhere to their treatment plans as they lack the confidence in their own skills to make positive changes to a patient's pain and function.

They feel trapped, incompetent, unconfident and isolated, a far cry away from what they expected life as a New Grad Physio would be like.

Maybe that sounds like you…

Maybe you haven't yet qualified and are reading this book as a student therapist but you've no doubt already heard many of the challenges and problems New Grad Physios have and want to learn how to avoid these problems and hit the ground running once you do qualify.

Whether you're a New Grad Physio, Sports Therapist or Sports Rehabilitator, in the early stages of your career in the NHS, private practice or sport, or even a student therapist working your way through your studies, this book is designed for you.

In this book I'm going to highlight the main issues faced by New Grad Physios that are stopping so many of them in their tracks. I'll show you the easiest way to build competency, enter the workplace and survive life as a New Grad Physio. I'll also teach you how to build trust with both your patients and senior colleagues to get your patients to adhere to your treatment plans, and show you the quickest way to get your next promotion.

These are all challenges faced by New Grads and challenges that you must overcome if you want to become a competent, confident and competitive New Grad Physio.

I have specifically picked these four competencies to cover in this book:

- **Competency 1** How to get noticed and gain entry to your first role in the NHS, private practice or sport
- **Competency 2** How to SURVIVE as a New Grad Physio
- **Competency 3** How to not only survive but THRIVE as a New Grad Physio
- **Competency 4** Getting your next promotion

These are the Four Stages of The New Grad Physio Competency Ladder and relate directly to the steps you must take if you are to become a competent, confident and competitive New Grad Physio. Without nailing these areas, your life as a New Grad Physio could well be a difficult one.

However, if you can nail these four competencies then you will THRIVE in whatever department you choose to work and have the skill-sets needed to get consistent, positive patient results and to fly up the promotion ladder faster than you ever thought possible. These are the four main areas New Grad Physios seek guidance on and are the main barriers stopping them from making progress.

Progression up the New Grad Physio Competency Ladder allows New Grad Physios to develop the **Three Cs – to become Competent, Confident and Competitive New Grad Physios.**

- **COMPETENT:** A New Grad Physio who is competent has the clinical skill-sets needed to understand their patient assessments, provide hands-on treatment and prescribe rehab exercises that take away a patient's pain and get them back to full function.
- **CONFIDENT:** A New Grad Physio who is confident can easily build patient rapport, gain respect and recognition from their patients and senior staff and can communicate their clinical messages well so patients believe what they are saying and adhere to their treatment plans.
- **COMPETITIVE:** A New Grad Physio who is competitive can stand out from the crowd, get ahead of their peers to get the jobs they want and fly up the promotion ladder faster than anyone thought possible.

Throughout your journey as a New Grad Physio you will be presented with many challenges.

Firstly, getting that first job in the NHS, private practice or sport can be very difficult. There are jobs out there, but I know many New Grads often take roles that they THINK they should take and DON'T pursue roles in areas they really WANT.

Being able to not only 'SURVIVE' but 'THRIVE' as a New Grad Physio is the result of being able to manage your caseload, understanding your patient assessments and being able to write and implement individual treatment and rehab plans.

Many New Grad Physios feel looked down upon by their patients and senior colleagues and that they are just seen as another young and inexperienced therapist. This is a massive problem because if patients see you this way, they will not buy into your treatment plan and as a result they won't get better; if your senior colleagues see you this way, they won't give you the respect, recognition and responsibility you deserve.

This has nothing to do with clinical skills.

It's all to do with understanding how to build rapport and trust with your patients and educate them in a way that they will go away and do every rep of every set of their home exercise programme.

If you want more responsibility and exposure to more complex and exciting patients, you need to be trusted by your senior colleagues.

Once these senior colleagues trust that you are competent and have the skills to do your job well, doors will open, and new opportunities will present themselves. You will be given exposure to more challenging patients, which will test your skills, but when you are successful with these patients, you will prove your worth; in addition, this will give you a much greater level of accomplishment and job satisfaction.

With the right guidance you can get promoted faster than you thought possible, whether that's progressing from your current Band 5 rotational post to a static position or even a Band 6 post; progressing from part-time to full-time in private practice or sport, or even transitioning from one area to another.

To do this you will need to improve both your clinical and non-clinical skills. Building patient rapport, communicating effectively with your patients and other members of the Multi-Disciplinary Team (MDT) and using the right language with patients are just some of the non-clinical skills you WILL need to get better at to become a competent, confident and competitive New Grad Physio.

Despite their importance, these skills are rarely even spoken about, never mind taught during university studies. With that in mind, is it any surprise that most New Grad Physios have poor non-clinical skills?

You could be the best hands-on therapist in the world and be able to write the best rehab programme ever seen, but if you can't build patient rapport and trust, or educate and communicate information well to your patients, then it is unlikely your patients will ever buy-in to your plan or adhere to your rehab; in turn, they won't get better.

Your journey as a New Grad Physio will not be easy. Let me put you straight… You are not going to read this book and instantly become the best New Grad Physio.

This book will highlight the most important aspects YOU must firstly acknowledge and then act upon if you really want to be become a successful New Grad Physio. It will require hard work, persistence and effort on your part. But added to the right guidance and support you CAN become a competent, confident and competitive New Grad Physio.

As a therapist you can be confident and competent instead of being overwhelmed, enjoy your job and most importantly help your patients to the best of your ability. You can be competitive, get offered a job in your desired area, rather than settling for just any job, and gain quick progress up the promotion ladder.

Never lose sight of why you chose this career path in the first place. You did it because you want to help people. You did it specifically to get people out of pain and back to the level of function they require, be that back to their occupation, gym, a hobby or interest, or even back to professional sport.

The level of function isn't that important. What is important is being able to facilitate patients to do what they want and to enjoy their chosen interests, without fear of pain returning. That is what we do as therapists; that is our remit for every patient or athlete we see.

We are NOT in the game to treat pain. Pain isn't the issue patients come to see us about. Patients come to see us because of what the pain is stopping them from doing. If it was just pain, they would self-medicate and go to see their GP. They seek therapy assistance because their symptoms (usually pain) are stopping them from doing something important to them. Being able to give a patient back that freedom, that choice of activity and the positive emotions that complement those activities is what we should focus on.

I'm guessing for a lot of you this is probably the first time you have heard this concept.

University teachings focus on pain and the management of pain and as a result have driven many New Grad Physios to forget what our actual jobs are as therapists.

Just understanding this simple concept means you are already well ahead of most other New Grad Physios that solely focus on pain, who direct all their efforts to the site of pain and give little, if any, thought to the patient's real reason they came to see you.

We will delve deeper into the challenges that you will face at each stage on the New Grad Physio Competency Ladder, but firstly I wanted to walk you through my own struggles and challenges as a New Grad Physio.

The reason I want to do this is to give the content of this book some context and show you why I am ideally placed to help YOU to overcome the challenges you currently face and how you can accelerate your own career, just like I was able to.

There is a big distinction between successful and unsuccessful New Grad Physios. The most successful New Grad Physios are driven to become better therapists and put the necessary time and effort into their own development.

But that alone is not enough...

The most successful New Grad Physios, those that get the best jobs, progress quickly up the promotion ladder and operate with competence and confidence have one thing in common. They all had a support network around them allowing them to succeed.

That is why I have developed the New Grad Physio Membership.

I want to help New Grad Physios, just like YOU, transition from university and into the real world with ease, and to teach you the content university didn't teach you – content you must know to become that competent, confident and competitive New Grad Physio.

Members within the New Grad Physio Membership receive group and individual mentorship to overcome their own New Grad Physio challenges.

Members include therapy students and qualified therapists who have taken action to bridge the gap in their university education and to gain the additional guidance they need to become successful New Grad Physios, Sports Therapists or Sports Rehabilitators, and achieve their own individual career goals.

These therapists are already well on their way to becoming more confident and competent practitioners. They realise that with some additional time and effort, and the right guidance, they will continue to make a big impact on the lives of the patients they work with on a day-to-day basis.

They have the reassurance of receiving help and support when they encounter a difficult patient or challenge as a New Grad Physio. This ensures they never feel overwhelmed or isolated and are never in danger of being left to their own devices to overcome the struggles faced by all New Grad Physios.

To learn more about the New Grad Physio Membership and how it could help you achieve your own goals visit **www.newgradphysio.com/start**

Just for clarity, in the book I refer to the New Grad Physio, but the content of this book and the New Grad Physio Membership is built for physiotherapists, sports therapists and sports rehabilitators.

Now on to my own New Grad Physio journey…

CHAPTER 2
My story – new grad to 'dream job' in just 15 months

From the moment I knew I wanted to become a physio there was only one job I wanted to do. I was very clear about what that was, and I am very proud to say I was able to achieve it. I'm even more proud to say I achieved this just 15 months after graduating.

It is not lost on me that many therapists will never attain that 'dream job' and get the opportunity, like I did, to experience the highs associated with their own 'dream role'. Many New Grads feel like that dream is a million miles away, but, in truth, it doesn't need to be.

I hope that reading my story will invigorate your own desires to pursue YOUR dream role and that this book will give you the direction and confidence to make that dream a reality.

But firstly, my career didn't get off to the best of starts.

In fact, I nearly gave up hope trying to get onto a physiotherapy degree course in the first place. I had applied during Sixth Form College to six different institutions to enrol onto a BSc Physiotherapy programme, but I received no offers.

Not even one interview…

Despite meeting the grades for all those institutions, I couldn't get on a course. I knew what I wanted to do and had worked hard at college to achieve the grades.

I'd picked a range of subjects that I found both interesting and challenging: Maths, Physics, Economics, and Sport and Physical Education, yet despite hitting the academic entry requirements I couldn't get on a course.

Things back then were not too dissimilar to now, and gaining entry onto a course was as difficult as trying to get your first job upon qualification, if not harder.

Additionally, at that time health study degrees like physiotherapy were totally NHS funded so students bore no financial cost via tuition fees. That made it very difficult to get a place, with demand so high and course places so scarce.

I had thoughts of giving it up as a bad job. It was out of my hands and I'd have to look at doing something else. I could apply the year after, the year after that, and so on, yet still not get a place.

It didn't help that the universities couldn't give me any constructive feedback on how to improve my application.

I later found out that I had in fact got to the final stage at two universities, the final 200 applicants, with 100 selected for interview. Both these universities chose those 100 for interview via random allocation i.e. they hit a computer button that removed 100 of those applicants. At both these universities that included me!

I probably would have felt less aggrieved and disappointed had I at least had the chance to go for an interview; then, if other applicants interviewed better than me, I would have been able to accept that. So not only could I not get on a physiotherapy course I couldn't even get an interview.

At that point I wasn't sure what direction to go in.

I was hoping to be the first person in my family to go to university but, at that point, it didn't seem very likely. I felt like a failure and very downhearted that I wasn't going to be starting my therapy training the following academic year and starting my journey to becoming a physiotherapist.

This was the career that I wanted yet it appeared I had hit a roadblock. I had contacted all the universities that I had applied to; most didn't even respond, and those that did didn't give me any hope or advice. As a result, I decided to take a year out of education.

I had played rugby from a very young age and used that platform to contact some clubs in Australia. I was able to contact a club in Northern New South Wales, who assisted me with finding a place to live and some work. I got my visa sorted, booked my flight, and I was off.

I spent the next 10 months playing the rugby season out in Australia, living with one of my teammates and his wife. The rugby was great, and I was living in a great part of the world.

A month or so after I left, one of my mates came over to join me in Australia playing rugby and he enjoyed it that much that he has never come home (We went over to Australia in 2005!). We bought a car and any free time that we had we spent travelling up the East Coast.

Whilst I was away, I had a lot of time to reflect on what I wanted to do. But I already knew what I wanted to do. I wanted to be a physio. So, I reapplied to start a physiotherapy degree the following academic year.

But you guessed it…

I didn't get a place… AGAIN.

Whilst again being very disappointed, I made the decision to enrol on another degree – Sports Performance Coaching at Leeds Metropolitan University (now Leeds Beckett University) through clearing.

Looking back now this was one of the best decisions I have ever made.

The degree itself covered anatomy, physiology, nutrition, strength and conditioning and coaching methods amongst other modules and gave me a great foundation for when I would finally start my physiotherapy training.

It was also during my time at Leeds Metropolitan that I met my then girlfriend, now wife, Sammy. She was a big help and gave me the support I needed to reapply to try to enrol onto a physiotherapy course for a third time. I was halfway through my Sports Performance Coaching degree but knew the only way I would achieve my dream would be to enrol onto a Physiotherapy degree.

So, following this degree and having reapplied, this time my application was successful, and I even had the luxury to knock back a couple of offers. This ironically included some universities that had knocked me back previously.

I enrolled at the University of Bradford.

I chose this university for two main reasons. Firstly, at the time they had the highest graduate employment rate for physiotherapists in the country and secondly, having looked around the facility and met the teaching staff I liked the look of it. In addition, location played a big part; studying here would allow me to move back home and commute.

I wanted to give everything I had, put all my time and efforts into the degree, to learn as much as possible and make the most of the opportunity that I now had. I had lived the student 'party' lifestyle on my first degree, but this was different. I just wanted to get my head down.

Fast-forward 18 months and my degree was going well; I was gaining good marks in both my academic work and on my clinical placements.

During the summer between my second and third year I had organised a placement with the Leeds Rhinos.

Earlier that academic year we were told we would have to organise our own elective placement as part of our clinical hours (part of the 1000 placement hours needed to qualify). The day we were told about this three-week elective placement, I knew exactly where I wanted my placement to be and I was really focused on getting it at the Leeds Rhinos. So, I got on it straight away.

I was conscious that a lot of elective placements fell around that same time period, along with other students looking to get shadowing experience or voluntary work during the summer academic break.

I knew I would have to get to work fast to give myself the best chance.

The main reason I wanted to secure that specific placement was firstly to confirm that this was indeed an environment that I wanted to pursue. I had a perception of what it would be like working in professional sport, but obviously at that point I didn't know.

What was it like working in that environment?

What were the good things about that type of role and that environment?

What were the bad things about that type of role and that environment?

I got my answer to all those questions and I absolutely loved it. I loved the environment and I learnt so much over the three weeks I was there; this only acted to fuel my fire to pursue this area as a career.

I must have made a lasting impression on the senior staff at the time as following the completion of my placement I was asked to stay involved with the club.

So, over the next nine months as I completed my final year studies, any day or half-day I wasn't at university, on placement or at work, I would be down at the club.

Over that nine-month period my involvement grew and grew; so much so that by the end of my third year I was in effect the unofficial assistant first team physiotherapist. I had my own caseload, I was planning and running pre-session rehab and mobility sessions and was involved in MDT and rehab planning with senior staff.

Unbeknown to me there was some restructuring of staffing at the club, planned to happen in the coming months, and as I later discovered I was being tested out to see if I would be a suitable candidate for a job.

It was tough combining my studies, placements, work and time at the Leeds Rhinos. In the week I would get up at 6am, commute from Leeds to Bradford and spend a couple of hours studying before my university lectures would start, working on my academic assignments, revising or preparing for my next placement.

I was very determined to get the best grades possible to give myself the best opportunity once I did graduate. I had the philosophy that I was in 'direct competition' with my peers, those studying on my course, plus other therapy students around the country, competing for the same jobs.

I worked out that if I was going against someone else for a job interview, I would be more attractive to potential employers if I had better grades both academically and on placement, and had additional experiences i.e. like the Leeds Rhinos exposure.

And whilst this was tough, I did it.

It was hard but I was really enjoying what I was doing. I was starting to see the impact we can have as therapists with the patients and athletes we work with. Whether that was in the NHS on placement, the sport exposure I was getting or private practice (I did some additional shadowing in this area), I saw therapists help these people get out of pain and back to full fitness.

I started to see first-hand how rewarding life as a therapist could be. The reason I wanted to pursue a career as a physiotherapist was because I wanted to help people.

Back to my third and final year I was getting ever closer to graduating. My studies continued to go well, even the dreaded dissertation! I continued to enjoy my placements and the marks I was getting, and I was continuing to gain confidence in my role at the Leeds Rhinos.

Looking back now, you could say those nine months during my third year at university were almost my apprenticeship, helping me bridge the gap between university and the real world.

During my final student placement, I completed a second MSK outpatient placement. Having had the exposure at the Leeds Rhinos, by this point I was becoming more confident with my MSK skills and used this placement as another opportunity to practice these skills and learn more about this area.

I had a great clinical educator, who gave me the right balance of support and autonomous working to allow me to problem-solve, and work things out for myself, but have that 'safety net' of support if I needed it. I obviously made a great impression as come the end of the placement I got offered a job. I was told a static Band 5 MSK post was due to be advertised very soon and that if I applied for it, in my educator's own words 'I'll give you the job'.

Once that placement had finished, I was back at university getting towards the end of my third year, taking those final exams and assignments and finishing off my dissertation. Graduation was not too far away.

I was also back at the Leeds Rhinos when I was able, gaining more experience, learning more from the senior staff there at the time and continually being given more responsibility. I told them about the NHS job offer and they were genuinely pleased for me.

The next week when I went down to the Leeds Rhinos, the then Head Physiotherapist asked to speak to me after the players had left. My first thoughts were that I'd done something wrong or said something out of turn. But quite the opposite. He went on to ask if I would be interested in a job at the Leeds Rhinos.

This was April; I didn't even qualify (assuming I passed all my final academic work) until May, and it would be another 2–3 months until I received my relevant accreditations and memberships (HCPC and CSP) to allow me to practice, yet I had two job offers on the table.

I had the offer of a Band 5 static MSK post, which, at the time and to this day, are very rare, with most static MSK posts being Band 6 or above.

I also had an offer to become the Assistant First Team Physiotherapist at the Leeds Rhinos, the club I had dreamed of one day working at.

As you might guess, it was a bit of a no-brainer for me and I accepted the post at the Leeds Rhinos.

I handed in my final assignments and completed my final exams and started work at the Leeds Rhinos the day after finishing university. As I didn't have my registration through, I was initially given the title of 'First Team Therapist,' with my role as the Assistant First Team Physiotherapist starting the day my registration was approved.

It was a roller coaster of a start. The team were mid-season and going well. So well, in fact, that only eight weeks after starting at the club I was part of the medical team at Wembley Stadium as we played Warrington Wolves in the Challenge Cup Final in front of over 70,000 people live, and millions more watching on terrestrial television.

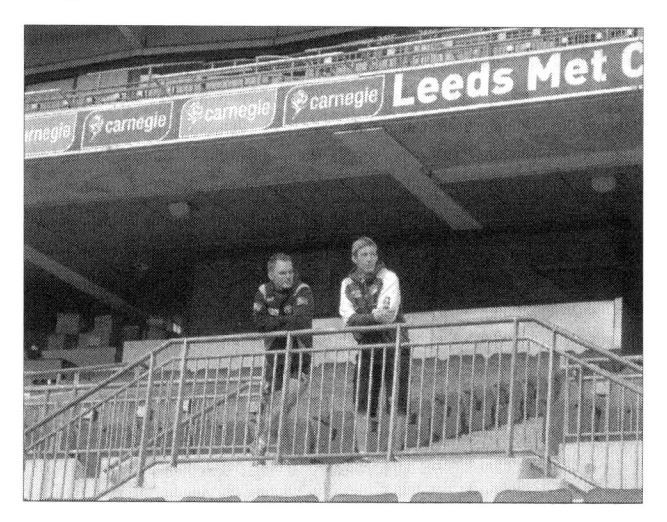

Having a look around Wembley Stadium the day before the 2010 Challenge Cup Final

But that early part of my career was littered with mistakes.

I remember many occasions where I found myself feeling overwhelmed and I realised quite quickly that there was a big disparity between the knowledge and skills I had attained at university and what I REALLY needed to know in the REAL WORLD.

I questioned myself as to whether I had jumped the gun and if this fast-paced, busy and challenging environment, working with a top rugby team, was too much for me.

I questioned whether this role had come too soon and maybe I shouldn't have accepted it but have chosen to ply my trade elsewhere before looking to pursue a job like this.

At times I certainly felt that I was out of my depth and I've got a couple of embarrassing stories for you in the next chapter to show you just what I mean.

The main reason I was able to overcome these challenges and to upskill very quickly was the fact that I had access to daily mentorship and guidance to help me navigate through the early challenges as a New Grad Physio.

I was fortunate to work with a great senior physiotherapist who gave me the support I needed, giving me the knowledge and skills that I hadn't been taught at university.

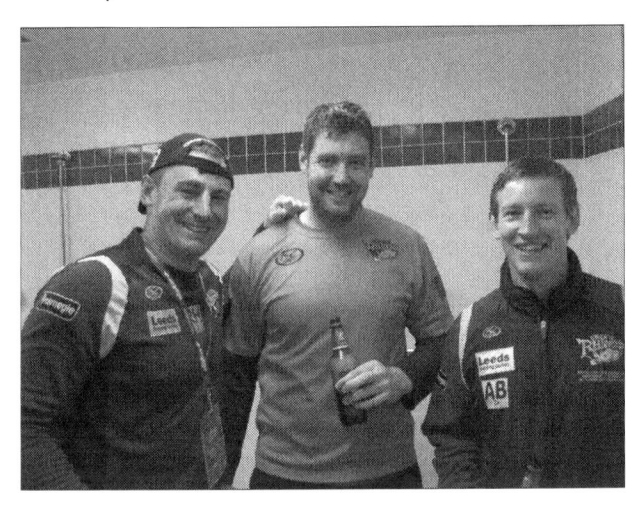

Strength & Conditioning Coach Rich Hunwicks, my New Grad Mentor David O'Sullivan and me after the 2011 Super League Grand Final

But I am aware this is a unique situation.

Most New Grads don't get this level of support, nowhere even close to this.

Most New Grads are asked to work autonomously, often feeling isolated, not having the opportunity to ask questions there and then. Most New Grads work in busy departments that don't facilitate a rich learning environment, like I was exposed to.

That supportive learning environment was the catalyst to my accelerated learning and progression up the promotion ladder so soon in my professional career.

A year after graduating the current Head Physiotherapist took another role, his own 'dream job', moving on to a job working in Rugby Union. That left the door open for me....

So just 15 months after graduating I had the opportunity to gain promotion and I achieved my 'dream role'.

I was promoted to Head First Team Physiotherapist at the Leeds Rhinos.

There is a bit more to this story, the specifics of what I did and the skills you need as a New Grad Physio if you want to attain similar quick progressions in your own career. I will cover these skills, in detail, later in the book and show you what you can do to accelerate your own career faster than you ever thought possible.

Fast-forward nine years and I have my own thriving private practice and work as a consultant sports physiotherapist, working with elite athletes from multiple sports, including being employed by the Football Association, working with England both domestically and internationally.

This gives me the perfect blend of working in sport, private practice and the time and flexibility to manage my own commitments. I can manage my own diary and prioritise things away from work, like spending time with my family, and allocate time working on other exciting projects, like writing this book.

Whilst the clinical roles I do are great, my biggest passion is the New Grad Physio Membership scheme and the rewards I personally get from being able to help New Grads at the start of their own therapy journey. I see the same hunger and desire that I had as a New Grad and I know with the right help and support they too can achieve great things.

I want to make clear I'm not writing my story to brag or showcase my own great journey so far.

I just want to make it clear right at the start of this book that with some hard work and determination, plus the right guidance, any therapist can achieve their 'dream job' whether that role is in the NHS, private practice or professional sport.

Don't believe these 'dream' jobs are exclusively for therapists who have been qualified for 10 years with plentiful experience in the respective field. I'm living proof that this isn't the case and many of the New Grad Physios I work with and coach are already on this same accelerated journey with the New Grad Physio Membership.

In the next chapter I will highlight some of the major misconceptions and mistakes ALL New Grad Physios make and I'll even let you in on some of my own embarrassing New Grad stories.

As you work through this book you will find links to additional BONUS resources.

These resources are completely FREE and are designed to complement the content of the book.

They will help consolidate the information presented in the book and delve deeper into certain topics related to the challenges you will face as you progress through the stages of competency as a New Grad Physio.

The first resource I want you to check out is my 'Success Planning Blueprint'.

You can get this resource here **www.newgradphysio.com/resources**

The 'Success Planning Blueprint' will help you set some career goals, individual to you, give you the direction you need and will in turn allow you to use the remainder of this book's content to be as specific as possible to your individual targets.

If you know where you are heading to start with, the path to becoming that competent, confident and competitive New Grad Physio is much clearer. Every effort, every decision, every intervention, is working towards achieving your goal and with this mindset you will progress faster than you ever thought possible.

So, hit pause on the book and check out the 'Success Planning Blueprint' NOW.

www.newgradphysio.com/resources

Once you've completed the short task, in the next chapter I will walk you through some of the main misconceptions and the biggest mistakes nearly ALL New Grad therapists make, to stop you falling into these same pitfalls.

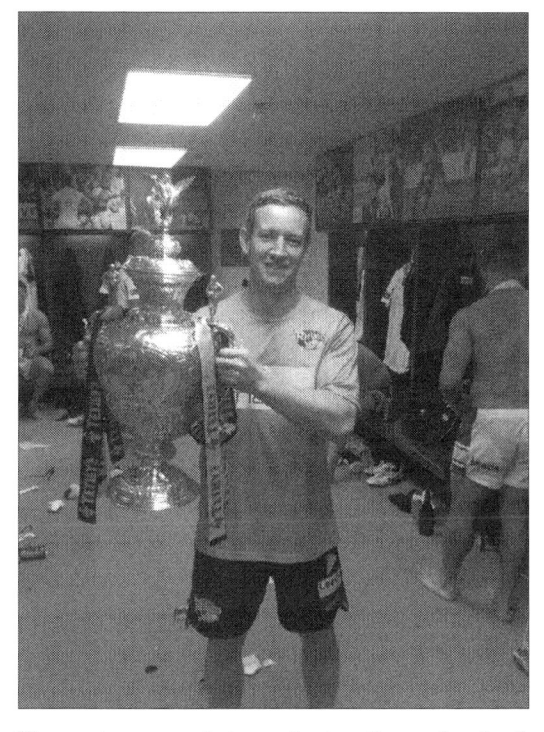

The customary victory photo after a final win

CHAPTER 3
The biggest misconceptions and mistakes ALL new grads make

So many of the New Grad Physios I coach talk to me about hitting the same roadblocks, the same challenges and struggles, that make their early professional careers unenjoyable and unfulfilling.

The catalyst for most usually occurs once they start to struggle with certain patients. Like them, you may have been able to make a positive impact on some of the patients you see, but there are some that you seem to really struggle with.

Sometimes, the treatment techniques and rehab exercises that worked so well with previous patients suddenly stop working.

Our university lecturers and the curriculum we followed taught us a simple system. We were taught that certain treatment techniques and rehab exercises fix certain problems.

But what do you do if they don't? No one prepared us for this.

No one told us that we'd be stuck in a treatment room, on our own with those feelings of bewilderment, not sure what to say, with the patient looking at you, knowing you are lacking the confidence about what to do next.

This is a real eye-opener for almost every New Grad.

It's the realisation that **there is a massive gap between what we were taught at university and what we really need to know to become a competent, confident and competitive New Grad Physio in the REAL WORLD.**

So why were we sold false promises of treatment and rehab techniques that should get patients better but that don't work in the real world? It's not that these techniques or rehab provisions were wrong. They clearly work for some patients. But they clearly don't work for ALL patients.

Never in a million years would we be able to study for three years and leave university knowing everything about every pathology, every clinical test, every treatment technique and every rehab exercise.

But that's the expectation. Once you are qualified your patients expect you to know everything!

Patients are coughing up their hard-earned cash for you to fix them in private practice.

Athletes (and the team manager!) are pushing you hard to try to get them back for this weekend's game.

Your NHS patient has waited weeks and weeks on a waiting list for an appointment with you, and they want you to take away their pain and get them back to the activities they enjoy.

No pressure!!

The biggest misconception made by New Grads is that some believe that once they have qualified that's the hard work done.

They think they've got their therapy 'badge'; they've got that certification and accreditation and as a result are competent enough to treat any patient who walks through that clinic door.

They also think it's OK to make mistakes; after all, you've only just qualified and all New Grads make mistakes.

But this is not true.

Your university studies have given you a great foundation of knowledge and some application i.e. our clinical placement hours, but once you qualify that's when the real challenges start.

I know how hard it is to navigate those early challenges as a New Grad Physio. These challenges are difficult for any therapist, regardless of whether you are a physiotherapist, sports therapist or sports rehabilitator.

Unfortunately for you, patients have the same expectations from a New Grad as they would expect from a more senior and experienced therapist. Our patients task us with helping them out of pain and back to function.

When we achieve this, it's great, and being a therapist is the best job going. But when we struggle, we become frustrated, lose our drive and motivation and sometimes even question if we are in the right profession.

As a New Grad I felt angry – angry that all that hard work I had put in at university had left me short. I felt that I was under-equipped and under-skilled to deal with the patients and athletes I was working with, and as a result at times I really struggled.

From the outside it might have looked like I had a smooth and effortless rise from New Grad to dream job, but this wasn't the case.

If I'm being totally honest, coming out of university, I probably thought I was better than I was. I had aced my exams and placements and had been offered two jobs before I had even qualified whereas some of my peers had scraped through academically and couldn't even land an interview.

I was told on numerous occasions that I was a very good student, hence probably why I was offered those roles even before I had qualified. I qualified in the summer and by the autumn the year after I was the Head Physiotherapist at the Leeds Rhinos.

From that day I knew that I wanted to be a physio – this was the job I wanted. This was my DREAM JOB. Most therapists may never get the opportunity to get their own dream job, but I had been able to do it, just 15 months after graduating.

This progression from student to assistant to head physio in just over a year was crazy looking back now. I couldn't have written the script any better myself.

From the outside, it all looks like rainbows and unicorns, but I can tell you it certainly wasn't!!

My first day at the Leeds Rhinos was one I will not forget.

The players had been on an army activity training camp the day before. During some of the activities a few players had picked up injuries. I was asked to look at a player with an ankle injury. He had jumped off a high wall into some water and having anticipated deeper water didn't control his landing very well.

I worked through my assessment and everything seemed to be going OK, until I got to my objective assessment. What I thought was going on i.e. my subjective history, did not match what I was finding with my objective testing.

This was the first time I had been left feeling baffled. I honestly did not know what was going on. The player asked me, the head physio asked me…

But I honestly did not know what injury he had. I couldn't make sense of my objective assessment findings and couldn't tell the player or the lead physio what I suspected was the source of injury.

I felt totally out of my depth.

I had graduated with a first-class honour's degree. I had scored 85 per cent plus on both my MSK placements and my elective placement in sport.

Why didn't I know what was going on? Surely I should at least have an idea what injury the player had. But I didn't.

I'll never forget that feeling. I can remember it like it was yesterday. I felt flustered and confused. I felt let down by my university teachings – why hadn't I been taught this?

I was in that treatment room, on my own with a player, and I didn't have the answers. I didn't have the knowledge and skills to diagnose this player's injury. I felt plain stupid.

Life as a New Grad had very quickly brought me back down to earth. And this wasn't just an isolated incident. Over the next weeks and months there were many more similar incidents.

Another time I was asked to co-assess one of the players with a foot injury. Not just any player, but the club captain and current international player. The head physiotherapist at the time asked me to palpate an area of the foot and identify what it was. I couldn't do it.

The player had a navicular bony stress response and, whilst I thought I was palpating the navicular, to my embarrassment I was on the talus.

I remember being asked to put a player in a knee brace and not knowing how to do it, or what settings to use. When the player asked me how long he would be in the knee brace for, I couldn't tell him.

I remember reading MRI imaging reports and having to google most of the text as it made no sense to me; some of the terms used I was reading for the very first time.

Additionally, reading post-surgical operation notes and having dialogue with consultants left me dumbfounded and overwhelmed. The athletes and patients I treated were having surgery, surgeries I'd never even heard of. I had not been made aware of these at university and had therefore never been taught how to manage them.

No doubt you have had some, if not all, the same type of experiences and associated feelings.

The early realisation for me was that I needed to learn more, and quickly. This acted as fuel to motivate me to be the best therapist I could be.

Now working with New Grad Physios struggling with the same challenges brings back these memories. I want to do everything I can, through the New Grad Physio Membership to help as many therapists through this difficult transition between university and real-life practice.

A big mistake I see New Grads making is to assume that this mistake-learning process must happen.

New Grads tell me things like:

'You must make mistakes to learn'

'It's all about trial and error'

'I'm new and inexperienced so its OK'

'I'll get it right NEXT time'

But this is NOT true.

If you want to become a better therapist quickly and accelerate your career, minimising the mistakes you make is key. You can quite quickly lose your way; these mistakes then become more frequent, resulting in you becoming increasingly frustrated and often demotivated.

These mistakes can sometimes be the difference between you being successful, being offered that job, being given more responsibility or gaining that promotion.

You need to show your current or potential employers and decision makers what you can do.

Would you employ a New Grad Physio who appeared incompetent, continually made mistakes, and looked flustered, frustrated and demotivated?

What if there was a way you could minimise these mistakes, get better patient outcomes and really enjoy what you do in the process?

What if you could learn what challenges and barriers you WILL face, before you even face them by learning from the mistakes of other therapists who have faced and overcome the same challenges previously?

Are your early years as a New Grad Physio ever going to be mistake-free?

Absolutely NOT.

But to create the best opportunities for yourself you need to be developing your three C's – Being Competent, Confident and Competitive is the only way to become a successful New Grad Physio.

Becoming successful is all about opportunity; firstly, knowing how to make your opportunity and secondly, being ready to take it when it comes your way.

Remember you are in direct competition with hundreds of other therapists for the same roles you aspire to, both therapists at your level of knowledge and experience and those who are much more experienced.

When you get an opportunity, you need to make a great first impression and be that New Grad that really impresses your senior colleagues. You want to be THE THERAPIST that has been earmarked as a future Band 6 or talked about in relation to a promotion to a full-time role in sport or that promotion in private practice, giving you an increased pay packet and responsibilities.

Regarding success – first we must describe what success is…

People talk about successful people like Bill Gates, Steve Jobs, Richard Branson, LeBron James and Wayne Rooney. But how do we know if they are successful without knowing what their goals are?

Answer is, WE DON'T.

We can't judge a person's success without knowing what they aspired to do in the first place. If the above people aspired to achieve what they are currently doing, or have done, then they are indeed successful.

Your success is about achieving YOUR goals and YOUR aspirations.

My career as a therapist has been successful.

My goal from the day I wanted to pursue a career as a physiotherapist was to one day be the Head Physiotherapist at the Leeds Rhinos. I was able to achieve this, very early in my career. But then my goals changed.

Once I had achieved that position, I could have put my cue in the rack, been happy and sat back.

But I didn't want to do that.

I didn't just want to be the Head Physiotherapist at the Leeds Rhinos. I wanted to be part of a winning culture and build a medical department at the club that would provide the best service possible to help the players achieve their best performances on the pitch and win trophies.

After all, a professional sports environment is about performance and ultimately results. I wanted to be part of a successful team.

I had a taste of that as the assistant physiotherapist at the club, when the team took part in the Super League Grand Final in 2011; plus some disappointments, when they lost back-to-back in the Cup Finals at Wembley stadium in 2010 and 2011.

But it was a different ball game being the Head Physiotherapist. Now I had to make the BIG calls, speaking with other staff including head coaches, CEOs and senior players and to manage other staff, making sure they were on top of their work and ensuring they continued to learn and develop.

If they made a mistake it would be me explaining it to the head coach!

My goals had changed and since then they have changed again several times.

Having had success as part of the team that went on to win a further three Grand Finals, a World Club Challenge, a League Leaders Shield and two Challenge Cups, which included the historic domestic treble in 2015, my goals shifted.

Full-time sport is very demanding on your time so I made further goals to set up my own private practice and attain experience teaching.

Over the next few years I built up a private practice and teaching commitments that allowed me the opportunity to leave full-time professional sport on my own terms.

Now I have a great blend of working in my own private practice, and consultancy work in sport and teaching, both at universities and the New Grad Physio Membership. I can manage my own diary, book out time for special events and book holidays when I want.

As I write this section of the book it follows on from a very diverse but great 'working' week. I have spent two days in my own private clinic, two days working with England at the Football Associations National Football Centre and a full weekday off work to spend the day with my family for my eldest son's birthday.

Too many New Grad Physios are wasting their time and efforts worrying about the wrong things – *What if this happens? What if that happens?* – rather than taking the onus on their own development and taking steps to learn the right things and to become a better therapist, upskilling clinically and having a plan to work towards.

You've already formulated your own goals having completed the 'Success Planning Blueprint'.

If you missed it, you can get it here **www.newgradphysio.com/resources**

Don't be like most other New Grad Physios who doubt themselves and lack the belief in their own abilities.

Maybe this lack of belief is perhaps not surprising given the shortfall in university teachings or the difficult challenges faced by New Grad Physios.

But, this doubt and lack of belief in your own abilities is stopping you achieving your own goals and will persist and result in disappointing patient results unless you act.

Just by reading this book you are already acting. This indicates to me that you are a proactive therapist, you value your own development and with that in mind I'm confident with the right help and guidance you will become a successful New Grad.

Forget about all the misconceptions, those previous negative stories you have been told about the challenges faced by you as a New Grad – the same challenges that will prevent you from working in your desired area or field.

Forget being told that New Grads are NOT able to fly up the promotion ladder and land those sought-after 'dream jobs'.

You don't have to follow the traditional university model. You don't have to complete your NHS rotations, internships, or shadowing before having the confidence to apply for a role you want.

I'm living proof that this isn't the case and in this book I am going to show you how you can overcome the challenges you WILL face as a New Grad Physio, give you the solutions you need to overcome the problems you will encounter and give you the best opportunity to succeed professionally.

Current members of the New Grad Physio Community are already securing jobs in the NHS, private sector and professional sport long before they were told they would. They are progressing faster than their peers and being given opportunities ahead of older and more experienced therapists.

So, forget these preconceived ideas and misconceptions and start your own successful New Grad journey. You don't need years and years of experience to gain that senior role within the NHS, in private practice or even in elite sport.

I hope it's clear, even so early in this book, that there is no reason why you cannot accelerate your own skill sets, get better patient results and ultimately get those jobs that you've been told in university are reserved for 'experienced' therapists.

If you are good at what you do, if you're able to get your patients and athletes out of pain and back to function, if you can gain the trust and respect of your patients and athletes you work with, if you can communicate well with your patients and athletes and the wider MDT team, then there is nothing stopping you attaining these jobs. Even if more 'experienced' and 'older' therapists apply for the same roles.

Provided you are willing to put in the time and effort to develop your skills, both clinically and non-clinically, then that dream job need not be a pipe dream; but a reality.

In the following chapters of this book I will walk you through the main challenges that you will face as a New Grad Physio and give you the solutions needed to overcome these challenges. I'll give you the solutions needed so you can experience success and become a competent and competitive New Grad Physio.

Some of these challenges may not have hit you yet, but by reading this book you will be able to identify what these challenges are and understand what you need to do to overcome them, even before they happen.

You might be currently facing these challenges and struggling to overcome them. As such the content that follows will be able to help you right here and right now.

Whatever your current situation, student therapist or New Grad, you will be able to take the information presented, use it to your advantage, progress past your peers and take important steps to become that competent, confident and competitive therapist regardless of the area you choose to work.

PS. To hear another embarrassing New Grad story of my own, watch my short video by visiting **www.newgradphysio.com/resources**

I'm sure you have similar embarrassing stories yourself. I'm sure you felt the same way that I did. But the best thing is… you don't have to continue to experience these embarrassing moments.

You no longer need to feel lost and isolated or look like that inexperienced therapist who lacks the knowledge and application to treat that patient in front of you.

There is another way…

CHAPTER 4
The New Grad Physio way

Having experienced my own challenges as a New Grad Physio, and having become frustrated watching other New Grad therapists struggle at the start of their own professional careers, I wanted to help, so I made the decision to launch The New Grad Physio Membership.

I had already helped many New Grad Physios overcome some of the challenges they were facing and found great reward in doing so, but I wanted to deliver a platform that would allow me to help a larger number of therapists. I wanted to deliver content that would upskill New Grad Physios and give them the support they needed during arguably the most challenging period of their professional careers.

The New Grad Physio Membership is the complete guide you need to ease your transition from university, helping you become a competent and confident therapist, who has the skills and feels comfortable delivering your clinical message to every patient you see.

As a member you have access to the New Grad Physio Membership Learning Portal (you will receive your very own unique login) where all the content is stored, enabling you to access any of the content whenever you want.

Each monthly teaching block will focus on specific areas on the body so at the end of that month you will have a complete understanding and get consistently accurate results with those body areas.

New material is uploaded weekly to the learning portal – material that you can digest in your own time and that doesn't take you hours and hours to work through.

I have purposefully cut the fluff and delivered material that gets straight to the point and gives you ONLY what you need.

New Grad Physios consistently tell me about their previous frustrations with some other online learning platforms. They watch a webinar for 1-2 hours or read several journal papers for the same length of time but are only able to take away a few bits of information that 'may' be useful.

That is why every weekly core content video in the New Grad Physio Membership is less than 15 minutes.

Time is without question our biggest and most important commodity. And it's in scarce supply.

Time is often the biggest barrier stopping New Grad Physios like you engaging in Continuing Professional Development (CPD) and your continued learning. Most of us have a lot going on: work, commute, studies, social life etc, and simply do not have the time to block out hours and hours of our week to CPD, as much as we would like.

But for just a small commitment of your time (15 minutes MAX per week) the New Grad Physio Membership will give you EXACTLY what you need to see rapid growth in your knowledge base and understanding, allowing you to take on any injury that walks through your clinic door.

But you are not just given material, like on a weekend CPD course, then left to work out how to implement this new material in your own practice. You are shown a system to assess, treat and rehabilitate your patients. Bonus modules specific to the subjective and objective assessments, hands-on treatment techniques and rehab planning show you exactly how to apply your new-found knowledge on your patients to get results.

Alongside the online learning portal, you have access to continued 24/7 support. You never need to feel on your own: you can ask questions about tricky patients or pathology and you'll no longer be totally reliant upon your senior colleagues for direct approval and help at work.

This 24/7 support comes via access to my PRIVATE FACEBOOK GROUP. Access to this private Facebook group is part of the New Grad Physio Membership and ONLY Members have access to it.

This group is the New Grad Physio Fast-Track Community. It complements the content in the learning portal and helps members develop their clinical reasoning skills, gives them access to help and support quickly and showcases additional bonus material allowing members to further accelerate their learning.

As a member of the group you will have the opportunity to post ANY questions you have. These could be clinical questions about those 'tricky patients' you see or could be questions about any parts of the content in the Membership site that you aren't totally sure on.

Weekly, I post a case study to the group that will challenge you to clinically reason and make sense of a patient's presentation. These are REAL life cases – not textbook cases, but ones I have seen recently in practice.

Presenting information in this way makes you think and reason what structures might be contributing to the pain experience and what interventions you might include as part of that patient or athlete's management plan.

At the end of the same week I post a video with the case study answer, talking through the patient's presentation and what management interventions were used, showing you how I have used the New Grad Physio Membership content to get positive patient results. This process gives you quick feedback and the ability to review your own answer and thought process whilst showing you how the New Grad Physio Membership content is applied with real patients.

Members also post their own case studies and 'tricky patients'. Maybe you have that lower back pain patient you can't quite make sense of, an ankle injury where the subjective and objective information doesn't match, or you just need some help and advice with another clinical issue. The group enables you get quick answers and support from other therapists and from me to ensure you never feel isolated again.

The group also allows me to identify specific problems and ideas that therapists are struggling with and these can also be worked into future New

Grad Physio content. This ensures your problems are dealt with as soon as possible and you have the confidence to treat any patient that comes through your door.

I also broadcast a 'Monthly Masterclass' live into the Private Facebook Group every month. The theme of this monthly webinar is chosen entirely by the members. Early in the month I post a poll with possible topics which members then vote on; the topic with the most votes is the one I choose to present later that same month.

I also post important new journal papers in the Private Facebook Group, allowing you to access up-to-date knowledge easily, saving you time searching for these papers yourself and saving you expensive journal subscription costs.

The New Grad Physio Fast-Track Community offers help and advice, giving you quick responses when you need them the most.

I add this content to supplement the core New Grad Physio Membership content as I want to make sure members have a clear understanding of the patients in front of them, gain confidence and clarity in their patient assessments so they don't fear that next 'tricky patient' and have the skills needed to take on even difficult cases and get successful results.

That is why the New Grad Physio Membership is much more than just an online course and why it gives you the support you need over and above what you would receive on a weekend course, and without the hassle of booking time away from work and expensive travel and accommodation costs.

You will no longer feel the need to continually keep running to senior staff to ask questions. You won't doubt yourself; instead, you will have the confidence to make the correct clinical decisions to help your patients out of pain and back to full function.

As a New Grad Physio, I'm sure you'll agree that moving from university into that first job can be very overwhelming.

You must deal with the pressures of managing your own patient caseload and deal with the expectations of patients and senior staff of getting positive patient results.

If you are anything like me, you have quickly realised the false promises you were sold in university about the treatment techniques and rehab interventions that SHOULD get patients better, but don't work in the REAL WORLD.

University didn't teach us that each patient and their injury is different…

They taught us cookie-cutter rehab templates and treatment techniques that the textbooks say should work…

But you soon realise that those 'nags' and 'snags', Maitland mobs, McKenzie style exercises or small knee dips don't work for most patients that you see.

As a New Grad Physio, the competition to get a job in the area you want, not just any job, but the job you set out to do and the job you've been studying so hard for, is fierce. You were never taught how to stand out from the crowd, differentiate yourself from your peers and give yourself the best opportunity of getting that role in the field you want.

At university we weren't given the skills and practice to be able to educate our patients. As such, we have no experience or knowledge about how to explain a treatment plan or basic pain science to a patient, or how to guide them on how many sessions it's going to take to get them back to full fitness or to know when it is safe and appropriate to discharge someone, without fear that their symptoms might quickly return.

Right NOW…

Do you have the competency and confidence to complete a full assessment and devise a treatment plan that is good enough to then ask your patient at the end of the session to hand over £50/£60/£70?

Do you have the competency and confidence to treat a patient in the NHS or in professional sport who has waited weeks on a waiting list and just wants you to take away their pain, or that athlete who expects you to get them back on the pitch in just a few days?

I know I certainly didn't when I left university.

Unfortunately, there wasn't enough time during our studies to learn everything.

I always remember one of my university lecturers proposing that a three-year BSc programme crams in five-plus years of study. Therefore, you can easily see why your studies are just a whistle-stop tour of your profession and it would be impossible to go into any great depth in one area.

This results in our knowledge being spread too thin, across too many areas, never getting to understand the complexities of the human body and as a result only having a limited knowledge base. That said, it's probably not surprising that so many New Grad therapists struggle so much as they transition from university and into the real world, working with real patients.

The New Grad Physio Membership smooths this transition by teaching you everything university didn't teach you, those missing modules, giving you the knowledge and skills to help real patients get better.

You need to have a clear clinical understanding of your patient's symptoms and be able to confidently get your message across regarding their diagnosis, prognosis and treatment plan.

The challenge you have is learning to problem-solve and make sense of these symptoms, building the ability to design an effective treatment plan, and choosing the correct hands-on treatment techniques and rehab exercises to get patients back to full health so they can enjoy the activities they want to do. Having the ability to do this gives you the authority you need to get that patient 'buy-in' and ensures patients have the confidence in you that YOU will get the results they want.

My background running my own private practice and working in elite sport has challenged me to find EXACTLY what works in the REAL WORLD.

Having progressed from university straight into full-time sport, alongside autonomous work in private practice, meant that I quickly needed to learn what worked with real patients, and what was going to get them better if I was to become a successful New Grad Physio.

If I didn't get the results, private practice patients wouldn't come back, they would go somewhere else, they wouldn't recommend me to their family and friends, and as a result I wouldn't get paid.

Within elite sport, failure to get the right results leads to loss of confidence from the players or staff, and would have cost me my job. Sport particularly is a very precarious environment to work in; it's a results-based industry, and if you are not getting the results, just like a player, you will be shown the door.

Over the years, my continued exposure consulting in other areas of sport, teaching in a variety of areas (undergraduate, postgraduate and the NHS), and opening and operating a successful private practice has continued to challenge my clinical and non-clinical skills.

That is why I know what works…

I know EXACTLY what gets positive patient results.

And having already helped many New Grad Physios overcome these challenges I now want to help YOU do the same.

In the New Grad Physio Membership I work with New Grads teaching EXACTLY how to:

- Identify what barriers are stopping you getting your desired job and what you can do to break these barriers down.
- Make yourself stand out from the crowd and learn exactly what employers are looking for so you can ease your path into employment.
- Set clear career goals and build your own clear path towards your own 'Dream Job'.
- Manage your own patient caseload, stop sessions running over and be

time efficient with your treatments, whether that's in the NHS, private practice or sport.

- Avoid overwhelming your patient by learning how to make sense of your assessments, understanding the WHAT and WHY of both your subjective and objective assessments and how to use this information to know what treatment techniques and rehab exercises to use.
- Select the correct treatment techniques to reduce patient pain and help them back to full function.
- Take a patient through a full and graded treatment and rehabilitation plan, from start to finish, knowing when patients are ready to progress.
- Build patient rapport and confidently communicate clinical information effectively including a patient's diagnosis, prognosis and treatment plan.
- Confidently explain to patients how many sessions they will need and know when it is safe and appropriate to be discharged.
- Gain the authority and trust from your patients to get full buy-in and ensure they adhere to your treatment plan.
- Build trust from your senior colleagues so they are confident you can step up to that next level and gain promotion
- Ensure you know what employers are looking for, so you can write a knockout CV, smash your interview, and progress up the promotion ladder faster than you ever thought possible.

These are the exact skills which allowed me to land my DREAM JOB, just 15 months after graduating from university.

The New Grad Physio Community is so much more than ONE course. It's everything in one place that will teach you the exact skills-sets you need to become a successful New Grad therapist quickly, to beat your competition and land the job in the field you've always wanted.

The New Grad Physio boosts your clinical education with modules university never taught you.

This knowledge ensures you continue to develop as a therapist at a fast pace, improve your skills and don't have to be totally reliant on the senior therapists you work with for support. Because, let's be honest, nobody wants to feel out of their depth and feel the NEED for continual support from senior staff once you qualify.

If you are operating like this, it's almost just an extension of your studies, like being a student on placement again, where you were expected to run just about every clinical decision through your educator.

Wouldn't it be great if you didn't feel the need to do this but had the confidence in yourself to make those important clinical decisions and were seen by your seniors as that confident, great therapist who gets patient results.

The New Grad Physio Membership provides that external support, so you don't have to burden those you work with on a day-to-day basis.

The content and additional knowledge you attain will enable you to get ahead of your peers and will even give you the ability to educate others within your working environment.

A big misconception of New Grads is that you need more experience to be successful. Whilst experience is important, as a New Grad therapist gaining knowledge is paramount.

You can gain all the experience you want BUT if you don't have the knowledge to appropriately assess, provide the correct hands-on treatments and plan patient rehab, then you WON'T be that successful New Grad Physio.

You need the knowledge, then you can apply that knowledge to the environment you work in, be that in the NHS, private practice or sport. This application then gives you the 'experience'.

Being successful as a New Grad or even as a senior therapist is ultimately about patient results and the ability to get patients out of pain and back to full health.

So, discard the misconception that 'experience is more valuable than knowledge'.

If you understand this simple concept and are prepared to dedicate a small amount of time to your learning to acquire new knowledge, then you are already a step ahead of the majority of other New Grads.

If you want to build your knowledge base, improve your assessment skills, improve your ability to provide patients with individual hands-on and rehabilitation interventions and have the utmost confidence in your delivery as a therapist then head over to the New Grad Physio Membership right NOW…

www.newgradphysio.com

Take that step NOW to stand out from the crowd, beat your competition and move towards getting the job you have always wanted.

The best therapists are the ones that TAKE ACTION, not wait for things to happen.

Even if the New Grad Physio Membership might not be for you right NOW, keep reading and even if you just take away some of the solutions presented in this book you will be in a better position to progress as a New Grad Physio.

In the next chapter I will highlight what you need to do to get noticed and secure your first role in the NHS, private practice or sport.

Even if you have already secured that first job, still read this chapter, as many of the themes discussed in it will still be relevant and will help you acknowledge potential barriers you are likely to face as you progress up the promotion ladder.

CHAPTER 5

Competency 1 How to get noticed and gain entry to your first role in the NHS, private practice or sport

If we look back to the New Grad Physio Competency Ladder at the first stage, you are at best...

'Unconsciously Incompetent.'

That might sound harsh, but at this stage, at the beginning of your therapy career **'You Don't Know What You Don't Know'** and as hard as the challenges might feel that you face right now, they are only going to get harder.

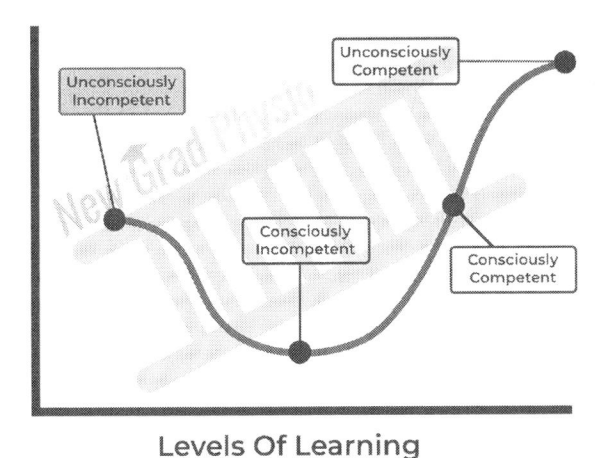

Figure 1 – New Grad Physio Competency Ladder Stage 1. Adapted from (Burch, 1970)

Whilst you are at the start of your career journey, many of the decisions that you make at this stage have a big bearing on what will happen later in your professional career.

The biggest challenge that therapists face at this stage is the unknown.

More specifically, the lack of awareness of what is coming and how hard the challenges as a New Grad Physio really are.

The main purpose of this chapter is to highlight some of the challenges that every New Grad Physio faces and give you some simple strategies to help you overcome them.

The First Competency Is – **Gaining Entry**.

This is the first big career challenge for any aspiring therapist and despite what you might have heard, it's not quite as easy as just sending a CV in and landing your dream New Grad role.

Even if you are already working in the NHS, private practice or sport, the content in this chapter is still of great benefit, as the strategies I share will help you on your way towards your 'Dream Job', not just your first job.

The First 'BIG' Career Challenge

Regardless of where you currently are as a New Grad, navigating the job market and progressing up the promotion ladder is no easy feat.

You might be looking at securing your first job following graduation or you might even still be studying and not yet at that stage of applying for jobs but have heard how hard and challenging it can be to obtain that first role.

There are jobs out there, but there is also a lot of competition.

This supply and demand for jobs doesn't really match up which makes landing that role ever more difficult.

But it doesn't stop there.

When I talk about getting your first job, I am talking about getting your first job in an area, or role, that you ACTUALLY WANT.

It's not about just taking whatever job might be available at that time and being content with just securing a job but entering the real world to a role that you will enjoy, and one that you will continue to learn from with genuine promotion options down the track.

Having put so much hard work and effort in during your studies, are you just going to accept a 'mediocre' role?

If you are anything like I was as a New Grad, you will no doubt have dreams and aspirations about where you want to be in 5- or 10-years' time. This is important as the career decisions you make early in your professional career can have a BIG influence on the direction you will go and what options might be open for you in the future.

We will get to that in a little while and I'll give you guidance as to how you can choose jobs wisely and give you all the help you need to enter your chosen job role.

But firstly, I need to reiterate, YOU DO NOT NEED TO FOLLOW THE 'TRADITIONAL' MODEL.

You DON'T need to spend 2–3 years doing your NHS rotations before deciding what you want to do.

You DON'T need to wait to enter private practice, assuming you need more experience.

You DON'T need to fear going straight into sport from university, even at the top level, thinking that these jobs are reserved for other 'more experienced', 'older' or 'better' therapists.

As a New Grad you no doubt have some questions about how successful you will be. These doubts are normal for any New Grad as you prepare yourself and adapt to life as a therapist in the real world.

But there is so much you CAN do, right NOW, to determine your career path, both in the short and long term, and give yourself the best opportunities, open more doors and gain employment in an area you want to work.

I see so many New Grads lose their way early in their careers. They have big hopes and dreams, they know where they want to work, they know their desired career path, but they hit a few hurdles and fall by the wayside.

They lose their motivation and drive and just settle for any job. This results in reduced job satisfaction and enthusiasm, and can block further career promotion options.

The biggest frustration for me is that for many New Grads this doesn't have to happen.

The choices and decisions you make early in your professional career have big implications for your future. That's the theme for this chapter – To help you make better choices to open doors, give you opportunities and the best possible chance to pursue YOUR dream job.

A Lack Of Intent Causes A Lack Of Result

You'd be surprised that most New Grad Physios don't know what they want to do and what they want to achieve.

When you really push most New Grad Physios and ask them directly about their career goals and aspirations most can't give you a solid answer. Is it any surprise then that most of these same therapists never actually achieve these goals?

Without the intent it is unlikely you will ever actually action anything and, even if you do, you won't persevere. If you don't know what you're working towards and the rewards that career would bring, why would you keep pushing towards it? You wouldn't.

Your motivation and enthusiasm will fade, and you ultimately give up, settling for a mediocre career, making every excuse under the sun as to why your dream career didn't materialise.

You kid yourself that you didn't really want that top sport job, or to lead an NHS department or open your own successful private practice anyway.

Or maybe you have a dream job in mind, but you don't tell anyone about this goal; after all, you might not ever get to this role and if you don't your career will be a failure. If nobody knows about your dream, nobody knows if you fail, right?

This lack of intent towards an actual goal even causes some therapists to pursue additional study i.e. Masters Level qualifications and training as they wrongly assume becoming 'more qualified' will make them more employable.

Others pursue further CPD, spending hundreds and sometimes thousands of pounds on additional weekend courses, evening lectures and other training, yet are left feeling more confused, unfocused and with even less career direction.

That's the reality of many 'experienced' therapists' career journeys.

As a New Grad you can avoid this, but you have a decision to make: you can either let external factors drive your career path or you can make a conscious decision to follow your own path towards your dream job.

Having intent and clear direction to WHAT the end goal is makes every career decision you make easy, as you know exactly how it is helping you achieve your dream.

There are enough clinical challenges to worry about, like making mistakes with your patients, missing red flags and feeling overwhelmed trying to make sense of your patient assessment, without making more challenges like securing a job for yourself.

There will be many obstacles along your way to becoming a successful New Grad Physio but with a clear plan and some guidance there is no reason why you cannot achieve your career goals.

Control The Controllables

I am a big believer in controlling what we can control and not worrying about things that are outside our control.

In a clinical setting we can screen patients and athletes with the view to preventing injury, but even with the best resources and processes injuries will still occur. An athlete might sustain a non-contact Anterior Cruciate Ligament (ACL) injury playing sport. As with every injury there are multiple factors that have contributed to this injury occurrence. Some of these factors are within our control and some outside our control.

Factors within our control would include joint and movement mobility, stability, strength, body awareness and control, the player's conditioning and training load and the learned ability to hop, land and change direction, amongst a host of other factors.

Some factors like the pitch surface, weather, number of games played in recent weeks (acute and chronic fatigue), international call-ups, bony morphology and general ligament laxity are not controllable, yet could have contributed to this player's injury.

If we haven't addressed some of the controllable factors, then we as therapists are part of the problem as we haven't given that player the exposure and robustness needed to operate at the level required.

With regards to your career and the job market, there are many factors that are outside your control.

- The number of jobs available.
- The number of years' experience you have on paper.
- The number of different areas, organisations or clubs you have been part of previously.
- Your degree classification.
- The location of some jobs.

These are just a few areas YOU CANNOT influence. And there are many more. So, what do you do?

Firstly, it is important to acknowledge all the challenges that you face, and then put a plan into action – a plan which ultimately discards the uncontrollable factors and gets to work on the controllable factors to make you as employable as possible as a New Grad Physio.

But before all of that…

I'd advise any New Grad Physio to test drive your dream job.

This is one of the most important things you NEED to do yet most New Grads do not even consider it.

Setting goals of your potential career path and your dream job is great, but do you know what it is like to work in that environment?

What are the pros and cons of your proposed dream job?

Have you seen what it is like day-to-day in that role and is it something you could see yourself doing and enjoying?

In short, is your dream job really your dream job?

Many New Grad therapists have never experienced and spent time in an environment like their dream job. Therefore, their perceptions of what their dream job is like and what it is really like may be very different.

Some of you might have been lucky during your university training and got good placements and the opportunity to spend time in organisations that you perceive to be the same or very similar to your dream role.

But most will not have had this experience.

That's why it's so important you gain access early so you can determine whether you are pursuing the right role for YOU. If you haven't had the opportunity to experience that environment, then you are just guessing what that environment is really like.

As an example, within sport, therapists often only see the glitz and the glam, the big games, the Cup Finals, winning trophies and travelling internationally, without understanding some of the downsides of that environment.

They don't often appreciate the negatives such as:

- Being restricted to when you can go on holidays – basically only in the off season.
- Missing out on important social events, family and friends' birthdays, weddings, christenings, weekends away and days out.
- The erratic work schedules that can change very quickly in sport and which mean you often have to cancel all the other commitments you had planned.
- The heavy workload, working day after day, after day, without time off. Within a few months of graduating I worked 42 days (7 weeks) straight, without a day off. (Some international tournaments and competitions can be even longer.)
- The short-term contracts in sport. Most often sporting contracts are time based; like a player's contract, they are not permanent and have a start and end date. Therefore, clubs have the ability not to renew at the end of a contract and leave you without a job. A contract like this can also make it much more difficult to gain things like a mortgage to buy a house or gain finance as you have a short-term employment contract.

And it's not just sport that this affects.

Have you considered 'on-call' requirements of an NHS post or evening and weekend work in your dream private practice role?

Would you have to move location to pursue your dream job? Have you thought about the expenses of doing so, for example the cost of rent, bills, transport?

Every job will have good and bad points regardless of whether that is in sport, private practice or the NHS.

What you need to do is gain access to these environments to gain a better understanding of what they are like, speak to therapists with experience in these environments and gain information i.e. the pros and cons of that environment. Then you will be able to make a much better and more informed decision as to whether your dream job is really your dream job.

Gaining experience of a sport setting during my own university studies was the best thing I ever did. It confirmed to me that I did want a role in sport and really fuelled my fire to pursue that role. It gave me direction and a focus that helped me stay motivated with my academic work and enthusiastic whilst on placements as I knew exactly WHY I needed to work hard.

Lacking a goal can leave you feeling lost, unmotivated and unfocused. Lacking the knowledge of the pros and cons of any working environment and not test driving it is DUMB.

Are you really going to spend all your time and efforts working towards a goal and a career you know nothing about?

Do you know if your dream role is really an environment you want to work in?

The only way to do this and to be certain is to 'TEST DRIVE' it.

So, how do you gain entry to test drive your dream role?

We go into detail in the New Grad Physio Membership as to exactly how to do this. This includes proven scripts and templates to help New Grad Physios overcome the challenges discussed above and test drive their own dream job.

These same techniques have allowed New Grads to enter, gain experience and even get offered jobs, some even whilst still studying.

These are the exact same methods that I used myself to get on the radar of potential employers and secure a job working in international football, despite having no formal background working in the sport.

So, how do you even get on the radar of your future employer? If you've been unsuccessful trying to gain an interview, or a job offer, and feel like you've not been given the opportunity to showcase your skills, then the guidance in the remainder of this chapter will give you a great start.

The Best Candidates Don't Always Get The Best Opportunities

Those that get the best opportunities are usually those that have done something different. To open doors and gain these opportunities, you need to start to think differently by putting yourself one step ahead of the game and in a position to forge a career in the area you want.

Most People's Favourite Subject Is Themselves

Whilst most people would hate to admit this, most people's favourite subject is themselves. And it's not just me that thinks this, there's research to back this up.

On average, 60 per cent of conversations are spent with people talking about themselves. This increases to around 80 per cent when communicating via social media.

So, if this is true, so what?

It's important because we can use this to our advantage……

It starts with spending time researching our intended future employer and building some background information, things like where they've studied, what they've studied, any research or special interests they may have or any material they might have produced.

This is by no means an exhaustive list but it's easy enough to carry out. A simple internet search will help you find most of the above without too much problem.

But why is this information helpful and what do we do with it?

One reason is that it helps you build your first interaction with your potential future employer. The likelihood of nailing down an opportunity by just asking for one is minimal.

When working in team sport I used to get up to ten applications per week, every week, asking for an opportunity – a placement, shadowing experience and paid work.

Due to the sheer number of requests obviously we couldn't accommodate everyone and as such we only rewarded those we considered to be of greatest value, those that stood out and those that showed proactivity and potential.

Just compare these two requests. One just straight up asks for an opportunity. This might be for a placement, a shadowing experience or even a job.

'Hi, I'm a recent New Grad Physio looking for an opportunity to come and spend some time with you, see what you do, as I want to follow and work in a similar field...'

The second starts with something like:

'I read your recent blog post on... ' or 'I see that you studied your MSc at the University of... ' or 'I noticed that you've got experience working with...'

And off the back of this, you can ask a question.

It's probably not too hard to work out which example is most likely to get a positive reply. Most attempts like the first one don't usually get a reply at all, or at best get a ready-made reply sent back.

The main difference between the two is that the first request implies you haven't taken much effort: you've just copied and pasted a request that you've sent to 100 other places. However, the second approach shows a potential employer that you have taken time and effort to find out a bit about them.

Making it personal to the person you are contacting is key. If you ask a direct question you are likely to get a direct response. That's the first step in communicating well and how you can start to build rapport.

What you ask is key, but just remembering above all else that most people's favourite subject is themselves will set you apart. By doing your homework or 'research' you can make it personal and open doors into a career you want.

But the real deal is the quality of the questions you ask because this will determine the quality of the responses you get.

If you have taken the time to research your intended contact, you will be able to attain enough information to ask an informed and direct question. The subject of this question isn't really that important. But it needs to be personal and relative to the information you have attained via your research.

So, what makes a great question?

Different situations, different people, different organisations will require different types of questions. As such it's not just about having a set of questions! It's about asking the right person the right question at the right time for the right reasons.

Asking an open question is a great way to gain positive responses, but these questions must have some direction. Open questions cannot be answered with a YES or NO response and as such they require some degree of thought and allow opportunity for multiple responses.

So, we need to ask better questions to get better answers…

Open questions must have direction. If the question is too open the reader might be unsure on what you are asking, or equally reply with a response that shows they have misunderstood the intended question.

Just compare these two clinical questions:

1. How would you manage an ACL injury?
2. I saw a recent video (link to video) you posted which showed some jump and land rehab you were doing with a player post ACL reconstruction. How might you look at progressing that drill?

More than anything, the first question is too open; it's far too broad. To detail a 6- to 9-month long ACL management plan is a BIG job and is NOT something that the respondent is likely to take the time to respond to.

The second question is very direct. It relates to a specific exercise and asks a simple question that would be easy to respond to. The questioner has even taken the time to post the link just in case the respondent is unsure which drill they are referring to.

The second question also implies that the sender has made a proactive effort to seek more knowledge, and that they want to improve and understand something in more detail.

Furthermore, the second question is something that might develop into an ongoing conversation, helping build rapport with the person you have contacted.

This is a simple thing and so easy to do but one that many aspiring New Grad Physios fail to get right.

So, before you send out your next email to a potential employer, ask yourself:

- Is my question open but direct?
- Does it appear that I have made some attempt to answer this question myself?
- Is my question worth answering?

If your answer is NO to any of the above questions, then DON'T send that email. A little bit of groundwork goes a long way and will help you open doors and create the opportunities you need to take those steps towards your dream job.

When the time does come to apply for jobs, your first role or your next promotion, you need to be ready…

Being CV Ready

We go into more detail about CV writing later in the book when we discuss the steps and skills needed to progress up the promotion ladder. But I thought it was important to address some aspects of this early on to highlight the lack of awareness New Grads have when it comes to their own CV and the importance of this document.

We don't get much, if any, help during our studies in relation to CV writing and interview preparation, yet when we get out into the real world these are the first big challenges we encounter. Most New Grads dismiss how important their CV is and how it can be the game-changer when it comes to landing that job.

We spoke earlier in this chapter about getting on the radar of future employers, but you will never get a job, or even an interview, if you're not CV-ready.

What if you saw a job advert this evening which closes tomorrow, but your CV wasn't ready to send? You have one of two options:

1 Send the last one you updated – this might bear little relevance to the job, doesn't particularly match the job specification and therefore probably won't get you an interview

2 Spend half the night updating your previous CV – being half asleep you miss most of the important content you would like to have included and as a result also don't get an interview

Or I guess there is a third option and you could not send it at all. In all three cases you're not going to get that call for the interview. You need to be ready and have a knockout CV ready and waiting.

You will need to make a few tweaks here and there for individual job applications to ensure you match the job description of the role you are applying for, but most of the hard work and the bulk of your CV should already be done.

You've already detailed and documented your strengths and presented them in a way that makes your CV stand out from the crowd and will get you ahead of your peers.

You have not used a template you googled and made a few adjustments to.

You've spent the time and effort to put together a professional document that will impress the person who is reading it and will engage them enough to want to keep reading.

Do you know that most applications rarely actually reach the person you think they should reach?

Due to the sheer number of applications in most medical departments, CV's are screened by HR personnel who work by a list of inclusion and exclusion criteria, with the successful ones progressing to the next stage. Only then might your CV be read by the actual person who chooses the candidates for interview.

If you're still wondering why you never get that call for an interview keep reading…

The Clues Are In The Job Description

Another big error New Grad Physios make is failing to read the job description properly. The job description is telling you WHAT the organisation wants from YOU and WHAT roles and responsibilities your job would involve.

Therefore, it makes obvious sense that the more closely you can match YOUR skills and attributes to the employer's essential and desirable criteria the more successful you are likely to be with your application.

No two jobs will ever be the same so you will need to modify your CV to suit. But, having the main bulk of your CV ready to go ensures you can spend time pairing your own qualities and qualifications to best meet those required by the job you are applying to.

A CV is a professional document and it may be the first interaction you have with an individual or organisation, so give it the time and attention it deserves.

It's not something you should throw together hastily.

A poor CV might be why you've been left frustrated with the inability to get your foot in the door of a medical department, hospital, clinic or sports club.

You feel disillusioned by the prospect of ever working in your intended area.

You blame other factors and reasons why you didn't get that interview.

Whilst you have other competing activities for your most precious asset – time – it is well worth setting aside time to write a knockout CV and might well be the difference between being successful with that job application or not.

Timing Is Key

Timing is something else to consider when you are looking to gain openings and opportunities in private practice, sport or the NHS.

A job advert will have time-bound deadlines; for example, the date to submit your application and dates for interview. But it is important to consider the timing of your approach for other opportunities such as placements, shadowing experiences and other potential openings within a medical department.

Any medical practitioner will tell you how hectic some weeks can be.

In sport it might be the week leading up to the first game of the season, the week where you have three fixtures in seven days or that upcoming final.

In private practice it might be the end of the tax year or either side of public holidays in the NHS.

These are NOT the weeks to contact people looking for that opportunity. Making contact during such times will heighten your chances of being *unsuccessful* so pick your time wisely.

One reason you might have got an unsuccessful response in the past might just be because of your timing; it might have been the right thing but just the wrong time. You need to do your research so you know what is going on in that department at that time.

The number of requests I have had from aspiring sports professionals looking for opportunities, but who had no idea of the time of season is unbelievable. It is not uncommon for people asking for a placement during our off season period when we are in the middle of our season. This just screams 'I haven't been bothered to take the time to have a look at what is going on at your club at this time.'

Is this someone who is likely to be given the opportunity to come into the 'bubble' of a professional sports environment and beat off the competition of others seeking the same opportunity?

Likewise, I have had requests from students and New Grads asking for shadowing experiences or placements in private practice over Christmas. Really?

I'll leave that one with you…

To close this chapter, I have another question for you…

What Is The Worst That Could Happen?

What is the worst that could happen if you set goals, work hard, yet still don't achieve your 'dream' role?

It's tough but a possible reality for some therapists.

What is clear is that if you take no action and have no intent and drive towards your 'dream' role then it is 100 per cent likely you will not achieve your goal.

So, do you have that much to lose? Most therapists never actually achieve their dream role so maybe not.

There are many barriers facing you and preventing you from getting the job you really want.

There are likely many other therapists vying for the same roles at the same time as you.

Remember the best candidates don't always get the opportunities.

The best opportunities are given to those that show the greatest desire to act long before the interview room.

There is so much you can do right NOW to make your path into your chosen area easier and to get your foot in the door in the hospital, clinic or sports team that you want.

Taking NO action is NOT going to help you.

A small amount of time and effort will increase your chances of gaining employment and landing that first role, in a setting you truly want to work in.

Entering certain departments and organisations is no easy feat.

But with some time, determined effort and the right guidance it might not be as hard as you think.

I hope this chapter has shed some light on just some of the areas you need to be aware of to help you enter your chosen field.

This is just the tip of the iceberg and there is much more detail and methodical planning needed to maximise your chances of entering your chosen field.

Don't accept mediocrity. Once you have nailed your goals you have intent. Then you need to identify what barriers might stop you achieving your goal and put strategies in place to overcome these challenges.

Then you need to stay ahead of the game, be proactive and get yourself ready so you are ready to take any opportunity that comes your way.

Time spent upfront, doing your research will ensure you don't sell yourself short and that you are ready to roll once that opportunity presents itself.

This is how you gain **Competency 1 'How You Get Noticed & Gain Entry To Your First Role In The NHS, Private Practice Or Sport'** and gain your footing on the first rung of the New Grad Physio Competency Ladder*.

*The New Grad Physio Competency Ladder has been adapted from Noel Burch's (1970) Stages of Competence Model.

Burch's Stages of Competence Model describes learners as falling into one of four stages: unconscious incompetence, conscious incompetence, conscious competence, or unconscious competence. His model implies that all learners proceed in a sequential, somewhat predictable, fashion through the four stages. At the unconscious incompetence stage, the individual does not understand or know how to do something and does not necessarily recognise the deficit. Conscious incompetence is when the learner does not understand or know how to do something, but now he or she recognises the deficit. Conscious competence is when the individual understands or knows how to do something; however, demonstrating the knowledge or skill requires concentration. At the level of unconscious competence, the individual has had so much practice with the skill that it requires little thought and can be performed while executing other tasks such as teaching.

CHAPTER 6
Competency 2 How to SURVIVE as a New Grad Physio

So, you've got over your first major hurdle as a New Grad and entered the working world.

If you hadn't realised already you will now: this is where the hard work really starts.

It's scary when you realise how different your experience was as a student and what it is really like working with real patients.

At this stage as a therapist you are working at Stage 2 on the New Grad Physio Competency Ladder and are **'Consciously Incompetent'**.

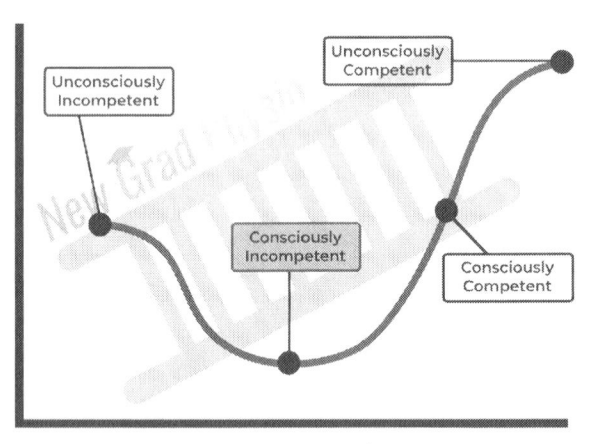

Figure 2 – New Grad Physio Competency Ladder Stage 2. Adapted from Burch (1970)

You now have an awareness of your missing skills sets and the knowledge gap between university and the real world as you **'Now Know What You Don't Know'**.

Previously, you were very much unaware of the challenges you would face as a New Grad Physio, but, at this stage, these challenges are happening.

This chapter of the book will cover **Competency 2** and show you **How To SURVIVE As A New Grad Physio.**

For most New Grad Physios this stage is a real 'Aha' moment. The penny drops and you realise what you know and what you need to know; the missing information and big knowledge gap between university and the real world becoming apparent.

The reality means that New Grad Physios at this stage feel incompetent and inadequate to do their jobs well.

Remember back to my embarrassing New Grad stories I told you earlier in the book? This was exactly the stage I was at then.

I remember those experiences – the embarrassment, frustration and anger at not being able to treat the patients and athletes I was working with to the level I wanted and the level I felt they deserved.

My treatment sessions felt rushed as I spent too long assessing and trying to make sense of my patient assessments and not enough time for any hands-on treatment and rehab to get my patients better.

I couldn't plan my time well within my treatment sessions, so my paperwork backed up as I struggled to learn how to manage my caseload.

When I did get to programming rehab, I lacked the knowledge to know what exercises to pick, leaving me feeling frustrated.

I felt that I was consistently chasing my tail without really making any great improvements with the patients and athletes I was working with.

Even when I did make improvements, if I'm honest I didn't really know what improved symptoms, as I often threw everything at patients, hoping something would stick. Sometimes it did; most of the time it didn't.

Moreover, I felt like I was falling behind, and I wasn't acquiring new knowledge at the rate I wanted to and the rate that I needed. Trying to overcome the above challenges left me no time to spend reading, learning and trying to keep up-to-date with the latest evidence.

I hastily booked on to evening and weekend courses only to find they didn't really have any great substance and in turn didn't offer any great help to overcome the challenges I was facing as a fresh-faced and inexperienced New Grad Physio.

The shorter treatment slots, the difficulty managing my own caseloads, the lack of time and direction towards my continued learning, and the added pressure and the expectation from my patients and senior colleagues made my life as a New Grad Physio tough.

I felt incompetent and inadequate to do my job and felt overwhelmed going into work every day.

I felt that I was unprepared and for that I felt angry and frustrated.

The frustration was mainly because I felt I was doing my patients a disservice and I was sure that there was a better way to work than the way I was currently operating.

The anger was because I felt university hadn't prepared me for the real world.

I felt my learning had stagnated, because of a lack of time and direction, and as a result I felt like I was falling behind my peers.

I knew I needed to upskill and upskill quickly. I needed to learn how to manage a caseload, understand my patient assessments and design and implement individual patient treatment and rehab programmes.

I no longer had the luxury of hour-long treatment slots or the luxury of my university lecturers or my clinical educators to turn to. The pressure and the expectations were tenfold what they were as a student. I'm sure you can relate…

In the NHS you might be working with 20-minute follow-up appointments.

In private practice you have the pressure to make quick changes to your patients' symptoms as there is an expectation you fix your patients, and quickly, as they are giving you their hard-earned cash.

Or in sport you have the pressure and expectation of professional athletes, the head coach and other staff to get your players back on the pitch for this weekend's fixture. In any example this is a far cry from our experiences as a student.

Nobody told us it would be this hard, did they?

What we were told and the reality of therapy in the real world are very different. When we first enter the world of work as a New Grad Physio, it's all about survival. It's about being competent and not making big mistakes with your patients.

It's the ability to be able to manage your caseload.

It's about starting to gain an understanding of what your patients' symptoms are telling you and having the knowledge to be able to write a treatment and rehabilitation plan.

Being able to do the above will allow you to start enjoying your life as a New Grad Physio.

After all, you've worked so hard to get to this point, you want to wake up on a morning and look forward to going to work. You've spent the last three years or so at university studying, preparing for exams, writing up assignments, and working for free on your placements for the right to qualify as a therapist.

You want to leave work at the end of the day with a sense of achievement, having enjoyed your day and having made an impact on the patients you have seen – no more feelings of anxiety and fear going into work. The content that follows will give you the strategies you need to SURVIVE as a New Grad Physio.

How To Manage Your Caseload

This is one area New Grads talk to me about every week. Even experienced therapists struggle to manage their time well and can't really manage their caseload effectively.

As a student you had the luxury of longer appointment times to spend with your patients. Now you might have as little as 20 minutes to assess, treat, give rehab and write up your notes.

It is tough…

As a New Grad Physio this lack of time left me feeling that I rushed my assessments and treatments, as I felt pressured to fit too much into my appointment slots. I was overwhelmed and, if I'm honest, I lacked clarity on what I was looking for during my patient assessments.

I was so intent on making sure that I didn't miss any 'red flags' that I was actually missing many other vital bits of information, details that I needed to be able to plan and implement a proper treatment and rehab plan.

So how do you avoid feeling overwhelmed and how do you deal with these time pressures?

How do you avoid feel rushed, even though your appointment time slots have been reduced?

The structure you were taught at university was modelled on hour-long appointment slots, but this is not reality. Additionally, most assessments were relatively generic. They were diverse in a way that would enable such assessments to be applicable to many different areas i.e. musculoskeletal, neuro, respiratory, to the NHS, private practice or sport. They were not specific enough or flexible enough to suit the actual environment that you now find yourself in.

To make matters worse, you are now probably seeing new pathologies and injuries for the first time, pathologies you weren't even taught at university, giving you an increased sense of feeling overwhelmed and frustrated.

The goalposts have moved so the way you assess your patients needs to change too.

You need an adaptable assessment that gives you the flexibility to ask the most relevant questions for that patient in front of you, not just the ones the textbook told you to ask.

You need to be able to manage your time well to ensure that you don't miss any important patient information during your assessments, and that you leave enough time for your hands-on treatments and rehab interventions to improve patient symptoms.

Such is the importance and challenge of managing a caseload, that I have devoted a full module to this within the New Grad Physio Membership.

In this module I teach New Grads the skills needed to be time efficient with their treatment slots, so they are giving patients WHAT they need, delivering the necessary hands-on treatments and rehab exercises to get them out of pain and back to full function.

The result is no more hours spent catching up on notes at the end of the day or feeling flustered and rushing through treatment sessions.

Gaining the clarity of how to manage a patient caseload and how to manage your time within a treatment session is key to overcoming the time-bound pressure of the real-life therapist.

Key to being time efficient within treatment sessions is understanding what your patient assessments are telling you; and that is what we will discuss next.

Understanding Your Patient Assessments

The main reason most New Grad Physios don't understand their patient assessments is that they don't understand why they are asking certain questions.

I remember as a New Grad feeling confused with the amount of information a patient would give me and I would struggle to sift through what information was important and what was not. As a result, I couldn't make sense of my assessment findings, often feeling like my subjective and objective assessments were completely different things.

I was told in university that my objective assessment should just confirm my subjective findings, but I was often left so confused at the end of my subjective assessments that I didn't have a clue what was going on.

My subjective and objective assessments didn't link together; my subjective felt scripted, almost robotic, and as result I couldn't diagnose sometimes even relatively simple injuries.

Added to this, I had a constant fear I might miss something sinister during my subjective assessment. I was therefore spending far too long on this section, leaving me with less time to use my hands-on treatments and to take a patient through rehab and the interventions that they needed to actually get them out of pain and back to full function.

I had an overriding fear of not being competent that I couldn't seem to shake off which left me with an almost constant feeling of uncertainty, worry and anxiety towards my job.

At times I almost felt withdrawn from the experience, distant from my patient, as if I was just going along with it.

Are you currently able to get through a full assessment, subjective and objective, use appropriate hands-on treatment techniques, demonstrate and coach rehab exercises, get your patient in and out of your clinic room, complete your admin and more importantly improve your patients' symptoms, all in as little as 30-45 minutes?

Given the above, would you be comfortable then asking your patient to hand over £50/£60/£70 of their hard-earned cash for the level of service you have just given?

If you can do all that as a New Grad Physio and be 100 per cent clear and confident that you have given the best service possible to your patient then you are truly special, because I have yet to meet a New Grad Physio at this stage of their career able to do so.

I certainly wasn't; I was a million miles from operating at this level as a New Grad Physio. Most experienced therapists, some with 10-20 years' postgraduate experience, never reach this level of delivery.

As a New Grad you have a perception that you just need more experience; you need to see more patients and more pathologies. That helps, but what you need is a time efficient assessment system that gives you only the useful patient information in your subjective history taking and an objective assessment system that is simple, easy to follow and is adaptable for ANY patient that walks through your door.

It's one thing 'practicing' on your classmates at university but very different once a REAL patient is on the bed in front of you. These patients have REAL injuries and need fixing. And it's your job to do it.

I teach my own system, the same system I use with world level athletes, as a bonus module in my New Grad Physio Membership. Once you see it, you'll realise it's nothing groundbreaking. It's a simple, easy-to-follow system that makes the process of extracting the useful from the useless information easy. It makes nailing your subjective assessment easy and the subsequent objective assessment that follows even more so.

You see, a great patient assessment is not a fancy sheet or the use of a few elaborate words. It's a simple system that is executed well, giving you the information you need to be able to make sense of your patient symptoms and as a result gain understanding on what to do next. Patients don't want some fancy assessment; they want clear and direct instructions and guidance to get them better. Whether you are 20 years' qualified or a New Grad, patients expect the same level of care.

Sometimes you feel inadequate. I know I certainly did as a New Grad Physio. You get that 'look' from your patient...

That look to say 'I'm not too sure I believe what you're saying'.

That look when patients see you as 'Young and inexperienced'.

Can we change how old we are and how many years' experience we have?

NO.

But 100 per cent of the time, a patient will not care when you graduated or how many years' experience you have as long as you take away their pain and get them back doing the things they enjoy.

It's all about getting results.

Most New Grad Physios at this stage of their career (Stage 2 of the New Grad Physio Competency Ladder) lack clarity about what they are asking when they work through their patient assessments.

They don't understand why they have been taught to ask certain questions and what the patient responses really mean.

They are seeing some new and more complex pathologies that weren't even taught at university, and lack the assessment skills to deal with these injuries.

They are starting to screen for red flags but don't understand what to do if a patient gives a positive response to one of their questions. They lack the ability to deliver even very basic pain science, making patients with positive yellow flag responses difficult to deal with.

Where do you even start educating patients about pain and how pain works; how do you explain hypersensitivity to any patient, least of all one with complex symptoms or chronic pain? The main priority at this stage is ensuring competency and the ability to operate as a safe practitioner.

Having a clear understanding of your assessment is key to gaining this competency and along with being able to manage your caseload, is a major factor in determining whether you will enjoy a successful working life as a New Grad Physio.

The third factor is the ability to design and implement a treatment and rehab programme with your patients.

How To Put Together A Patient Treatment and Rehab Plan

The third biggest factor stopping New Grad Physios from gaining successful patient results is their inability to put together a patient treatment and rehab plan.

You've probably already been stumped when a patient has put you on the spot and asked you something like this...

- *How many reps, sets and how many times should I do this rehab?*
- *How many sessions will I need?*
- *When will I be able to go back to work?*
- *When is it safe for me to start running again?*

These are questions we get asked daily by our patients. I remember as a New Grad I didn't know what to say. I remember trying to fluff some sort of reply, skirt round the question and give a response that didn't really answer the original patient question. I did that because I didn't really know. I didn't know why I was giving patients 3 x 10 of an exercise, or how many sessions a patient would need. I was guessing when I told patients when they should expect to get back to work or back to activities like running.

I also didn't have the conviction to know when I should next book that patient back in, or equally know when to discharge them, confident that they could go back to their previous level of function without fear that their symptoms might return.

I couldn't answer any of these questions because I didn't have a treatment and rehab planning system. I didn't know how to progress a patient through a treatment plan with the confidence that they were ready to move on. I didn't have the conviction and clarity with my treatment and rehab planning to know what stages or milestones patients needed to hit before I progressed them.

If a patient asked me what the stages of their proposed treatment plan were i.e. how I was going to take them from their current injury state back to full health, I couldn't give them a clear plan. If I wasn't clear myself about what I was delivering, if I didn't have the belief in my own treatment system, then how could I expect patients to believe in what I was telling them?

If I'm being completely honest I have only in the last few years nailed my own treatment and rehab planning system.

It's taken me close to 10 years to do so and even now I'm constantly updating it. But now I have absolute clarity about the steps I need to take every patient through to get them out of pain and back to full function. Above all else, I have the confidence to know that when they do return to activity, they will not break down again.

Having a system gives me the understanding about what I am delivering to each patient I see, and what to do if something isn't going to plan. Occasionally patients might not improve at the speed I expect them to. Having a system allows me to double check if I've missed something – maybe they need to regress for a short period to the previous stage.

If you cannot plan a basic treatment and rehab programme, then can you really say with conviction that you are progressing a patient as quickly as you should be? Do you know if you are holding a patient back or indeed progressing them too quickly and running the risk of causing their symptoms to return?

Before I nailed this process, I felt inadequate, and that I was failing my patients. I lacked clarity about what I was doing and as such I couldn't communicate a treatment plan to my patients. This inability to communicate led to my patients losing trust and confidence about what I was saying and reduced my authority as a therapist. They just saw me as that young and inexperienced therapist.

The three factors discussed in this chapter – managing a caseload, understanding your patient assessments and how to put together a patient treatment and rehab plan are the cornerstones to surviving as a New Grad Physio.

These factors are the cornerstones to developing **Competency 2** and **'How To SURVIVE As A New Grad Physio'.** These are the three key areas that New Grad Physios struggle with the most and hence why I teach these three topics as individual bonus modules during Stage 2 of my New Grad Physio Membership.

I wanted to close this chapter with just one more problem that New Grads commonly experience.

Falling Behind On Learning

Almost every New Grad I have coached has talked about how they struggle to integrate CPD into their working week once they graduate. Once they start working, they find it hard to keep up to date with the current knowledge and evidence and feel like they are falling behind their peer group.

Whilst once studious at university, they are no longer reading and learning, and as a result they feel like they are missing out on key information and key advances in the sciences. They feel that their learning and development has stagnated, and may even feel guilty that they are no longer able to prioritise their learning.

It's a tough scenario to be in. You acknowledge the knowledge gap between university and the real world, yet you are unable to access, find the time, or have the direction needed to upskill.

You no longer have access to continuing education material, like journals and articles, like you had at university. You no longer have that university lecturer telling you what to read or a module handbook with 'recommended reading lists'. You are unsure what CPD to pursue.

Some weekend courses can set you back anything up to £700-£800 and that's before any travel or accommodation costs.

New Grads talk to me about feeling lost and unsure about what to learn, with many feeling they have previously wasted their time and money on the wrong type of education.

I personally have spent £1000s on CPD courses and whilst at the time I thought they were useful I barely use most of the content now.

I used to find I'd go on a new course, learn new material and be excited to use it once I was back in clinic the next week. I'd use some of the new material, but as the weeks went on it would slowly fade away to the point that I wouldn't be using any of it at all. The problem was, it didn't fit into a system.

Most courses centre around a specific treatment method, pathology or someone's opinion about how to manage a specific injury or body area. What none of these courses ever do is show you how to integrate their new material into your own system, your own way of doing things, and that is why it is so hard to integrate and apply it.

Once you graduate, whilst you do lose that learning support network from your university it isn't as hard as you think to stay on top of your learning as a New Grad Physio. As busy as your working week may seem, you can still find time to stop stagnating and fill the knowledge gaps you need to.

Previously you've not been able to do this because you simply have been trying to consume the wrong type of material. Given the constraints on your time at work and the desire to have some sort of social life, you need short, sharp, concise content.

You need content that cuts the fluff and gives you the knowledge and skills you need to become that successful New Grad Physio.

You need a 'system' rather than just individual skill sets, and you need direction on what is important and what is not, saving you both time and money.

You need content to be accessible and support available whenever you need it. You need to be able to access this content wherever you are: at home, in the clinic, in the hospital or at the sports club.

You need a format that allows you to receive continued individual help and support to develop your clinical and non-clinical skills and guide your career, not just short-lived content that a weekend course or evening lecture delivers.

Above all else, you need content that is specifically made for you, a New Grad Physio, and content that addresses the actual problems you are facing right now. Content delivered this way means that you have the support you need, and you will never feel lost, isolated and on your own.

There are already New Grad Physios receiving content specific to the challenges you are currently facing – content you can find the time to consume. It includes a support network of fellow New Grads and experts to help you become a competent, confident and competitive New Grad Physio.

To learn more visit **www.newgradphysio.com**

PS. I've also put together a 'Survival Guide', summarising the main challenges you will face as a New Grad Physio and how to SURVIVE these challenges. You can access this resource completely FREE at **www.newgradphysio.com/resources**

CHAPTER 7
Competency 3 How to not only survive but THRIVE as a New Grad Physio

Having got over the realisation of how hard life as a New Grad really is, you've put in the hard work and, if you've had the right guidance and support, you will have started to find your feet as a New Grad Physio.

This progression moves us from Stage 2 'Consciously Incompetent' to Stage 3 **'Consciously Competent'** on the New Grad Physio Competency Ladder.

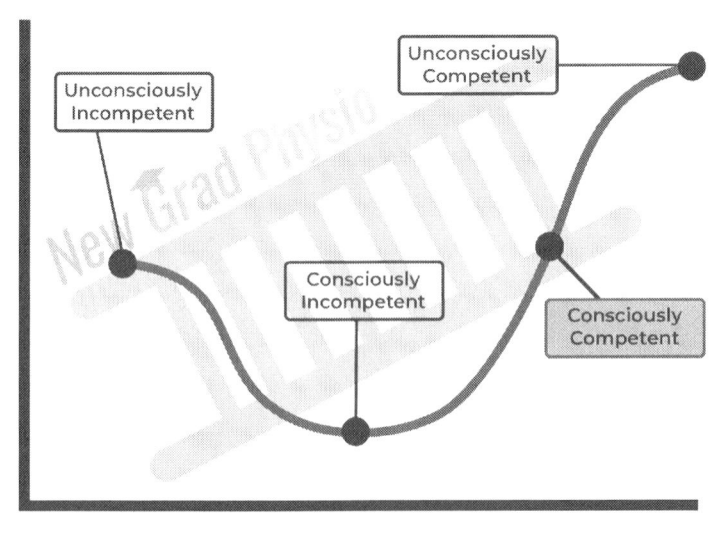

Figure 3 – New Grad Physio Competency Ladder Stage 3. Adapted from (Burch, 1970).

At this stage New Grad Physios are starting to build proficiency in their practice and many basic skills are becoming more automatic. But as you progress, more responsibility, more pressure and more expectation from both your patients and your senior colleagues, falls at your door.

The skills we cover in this chapter are largely non-clinical but are imperative if you are to continue your successful path toward a higher-level role, your next promotion, increased responsibility, an increased salary and increased job satisfaction.

Once I got a taste of success as a New Grad Physio I wanted more. Once I had found my feet, I wanted to progress.

Only a few months in to working as the Assistant First Team Physio at the Leeds Rhinos, I aspired to move up the promotion ladder and become the Head Physiotherapist.

I wanted to be the one leading the department, mentoring other junior physios and covering the big games. I wanted the pressure and the added expectations the role would bring. Whilst I knew how big a challenge that role would be, it excited me.

I remember having a meeting with my mentor, the then Head Physiotherapist, and telling him this. In short, I was telling him I wanted his job! He was great and helped me build a plan to achieve this.

Over the next 12 months he taught me everything that I would need to know so I was ready to make that step up. These are the exact same skills that I am going to cover in this chapter.

As much as it was about becoming better at my assessments, my hands-on treatments and my rehab planning, it was about learning how to communicate and build rapport with senior staff, including head coaches and CEOs, how to gain the respect and trust of the senior players and how to get the players to see me as the senior authority figure at the club.

This chapter of the book will cover **Competency 3** and show you '**How To Not Only Survive But THRIVE As A New Grad Physio**'.

The Reality…

At Stage 3 of the New Grad Physio Competency Ladder, therapists are starting to work at a level aligned to being **'Consciously Competent'.**

The current reality at this stage is New Grads who are starting to get some wins with their patients, but struggle with more complex patients, frustrated when symptoms return.

Whilst you may be building some new knowledge, the application of this knowledge is poor.

This stage is all about building proficiency.

A therapist at this stage would be someone working at Band 5 level in the NHS, entry level in a private practice role or a part-time (academy level) sports role.

A day in the life of a therapist at this level includes simple caseloads and limited 'real' responsibility – lack of input in Multi-Disciplinary Team (MDT) meetings and decision-making.

Therapists struggle to apply the knowledge they have, and, even though they are getting more experience and seeing a greater number of patients, they feel they are still not getting the trust and respect they deserve from their patients and senior colleagues.

This lack of trust is causing patients to not adhere to their treatment plans and as a result it is making it increasingly difficult to achieve positive patient results.

This leads to an increased feeling of being overwhelmed and an overriding feeling of frustration that patients and senior colleagues still see you as that young and inexperienced therapist.

I remember as a New Grad Physio trying to earn the trust and respect of paying private practice customers and top-level rugby players. Aside from upskilling in respect to my clinical skills, I knew that I needed to learn how to get the patients and athletes I was working with to buy into what I was saying.

I needed to learn how to gain the respect and trust of the players and private patients I was working with, alongside the senior staff I was working under.

The main reason the application of my knowledge was poor was the fact that I lacked the ability to build rapport and communicate effectively with both my patients and senior staff.

New Grad Physios right now tell me the same thing.

It resonates with me as I can remember so well the same challenges I had as a New Grad.

I also know that unless you learn how to build rapport and communicate well with your patients and senior colleagues you will never attain the trust and respect you need.

This lack of trust and belief in you as a therapist results in poor patient adherence to your treatment plans and in turn means patients don't get better.

Additionally, the same lack of trust will mean that your seniors don't give you more responsibilities, they don't see you as a New Grad who is worth supporting and developing and they don't see you as a therapist worthy of that next promotion.

Therefore, the main theme of this chapter is to show you how to communicate and build trust and rapport with your patients, so they adhere to your treatment plans, as well as with senior colleagues.

Getting Patients To Do What We Want Them To Do

We give patients advice and a home exercise programme for a reason.

We have assessed them, found the problems and given them the solutions (i.e. their home exercise programme) to get them better. Patients want to get better, but why is it that some patients don't trust what you are saying and don't adhere to your treatment plan?

Whatever domain you work in, whether that's a hospital, private or sports setting, getting patients or athletes to do what you want them to do is challenging.

We advise and prescribe exercises on the basis these will aid that person to improve their symptoms and/or dysfunctions. Some take our advice on board, crack on with their prescribed rehab and symptoms improve. Other patients don't engage with the rehab and, as a result, symptoms don't improve.

We have based our rehab provision on evidence-based practice and experience to try and help these people, therefore it can be frustrating when they don't engage.

But why don't they engage?

I remember patients saying things to me as a New Grad like:

'My symptoms are similar, but I haven't really done my rehab as much as should.'

'I had a really busy week and didn't really find the time to do my rehab.'

They might even try being nice to you by saying something like:

'I wasn't too sure about how to do my rehab exercises properly, so I just didn't do them.'

In all the above examples they haven't done their home exercise programme because they don't value it. They haven't bought into your treatment plan and as a result haven't completed their rehab.

Underlying everything we do as therapists is getting our patients on board. If we are unable to do that, patients will not have clarity or understanding about what they are doing and why they are doing it. As a result, they won't do it.

And if patients don't adhere to your treatment plan, it's highly likely their symptoms are not going to improve.

You can write the best treatment plan in the world but if your patient won't do it, it is not worth the paper it is written on.

I know as a New Grad I lacked the confidence in the delivery of what I was telling patients to do. Some of this stemmed from my lack of confidence with my assessment skills and being unsure of my diagnosis and prognosis skills.

It was also the result of not having a system and not knowing exactly what steps I needed to take each patient through to get them totally out of pain and back to full function, without the fear that their symptoms would return.

But a large part of my lack of confidence in my delivery was non-clinical.

I lacked the ability to communicate information effectively to my patients.

I struggled to build rapport, to put patients at ease, and, when it came to delivering my assessment findings or explaining my proposed treatment plan, I communicated this information poorly.

I could see in my patients' faces and by their body language that they weren't 100 per cent on board with my treatment plan.

Even when I had nailed my assessment and had a clear treatment plan, my poor delivery of this information was causing poor patient adherence to the plan.

I was left feeling frustrated as I couldn't implement what I planned; plus it's not a great feeling when patients don't trust and believe what you are saying.

I used to blame the patients. I used to just think it was their problem. I was giving them help and advice and they were consciously choosing not to follow it, therefore, it was their problem.

How did they expect to get better if they weren't willing to do their home exercise programme?

But looking back now, I know the main issue was me.

It was a direct result of my poor communication and delivery skills.

I couldn't present information in the correct way so that patients both understood what I was saying and had a clear plan as to why the rehab I was prescribing was going to help them get back to what they wanted to do, be that playing rugby, gardening or running.

So how do we get our patients to do what we want them to do?

I believe the main issue why patients don't adhere to their treatment plan relates to trust.

The level of trust between the therapist and the patient is imperative for engagement in rehabilitation. Without it, we are going to struggle to get buy-in to our programmes and ultimately this makes our goal of patient or athlete improvement much more difficult.

There are two main reasons why trust might be missing between you as a New Grad Physio and your patient.

Firstly, the patient must believe what we say and have faith in the programme of action we provide.

This boils down to patients believing you are competent in what you are doing.

Your patients need to believe you have the necessary skill-sets to be able to help them in their quest for improvement, to get them out of pain and back to function.

If they don't believe you have the necessary skills and knowledge, then why would they trust what you are saying and why would they engage?

Why would they buy-in, complete their rehab, and complete every rep of every set of each rehab exercise you prescribed? They won't and they don't, unless they believe we know what we are talking about and are a competent therapist.

Secondly, a lack of trust can prevail if patients believe we don't share the common goal with them of being 100 per cent on board with helping them get better.

When you are with a patient you need to make them feel that THEY are the most important person in the world at that time.

They need to feel that you are giving them 100 per cent attention and effort and have the desire to want to get them back up to speed as quickly as possible.

I see this often in private practice whereby patients often feel previous therapists have kept hold of them for too long.

I see a lot of private practice patients who were left unsatisfied with their previous level of care.

When questioned they commonly describe that they thought their previous therapists saw them either too much or for too long, some even questioning whether they had a superior financial motive that superseded the patient's symptom improvement motive.

If patients don't think we have the minerals (competency) in what we practice and if they believe we don't share the same motives (patient improvement and patient satisfaction) then patient outcomes are more likely to prove unsuccessful.

Building trust or buy-in is a complete necessity to help you as a New Grad Physio build a relationship with the patients and athletes you work with.

This is the only way that you will start to get patients better and not just survive but start to thrive as a New Grad Physio.

Looking a bit more closely into communication, it is important that we package what we are saying correctly.

As a medical professional we will deal with a variety of different people and, whilst the message might be the same, the way this message is delivered will be different for each person you interact with.

In this next section I will highlight why you need to explain things the right way and ensure your message is received in the way that you want it to be received.

Explain Things In The Right Way

Giving an explanation is person-specific – what you say is directly related to who you are talking to.

Regardless of the area you work, whether NHS, private practice or sport, you need to be able to adapt your message so that the person receiving it can understand.

A conversation with a consultant will be different from one with a fellow therapist, a patient or an athlete.

You will explain things differently, in different levels of detail; your language and terminology will be different, even your tone and body language may need to change to ensure accurate and effective delivery of your information.

The information I present within a sports setting is a great example.

I may communicate medical information very differently to a fellow practitioner than I would to an athlete.

I am more likely to use layman's terms as opposed to medical terms to explain a diagnosis to an athlete. On the flip side, a fellow medic will understand medical terminology and as such I am likely to use such language. The message is the same; it's the same information, but it is packaged differently.

To take that a step further, you may even need to alter how you address the same populations. For example, you may have two athletes who sustain the same injury although you might explain the diagnosis very differently.

Athlete A might need to be well informed, and want to know the structures at fault and the mechanics behind what the job of those structures is; he may need an in-depth explanation as to how your rehab programme is going to fix them and keep them injury-free in the future.

Athlete B, on the other hand, might only want to know how many games he is going to miss and when he is likely to be back playing.

In the case of Athlete A, I have found the use of timelines to be very effective. The timelines show the athlete what they will be required to do week to week, day to day, highlighting certain rehab milestones e.g. remove brace or commence running. Such detail keeps those players informed throughout the rehab process. Such detail might not be necessary for Athlete B.

Tailoring what we say to the correct person is key, primarily to give them the correct level of information they require at that time point.

Giving the correct level of information is so important; giving someone too much or indeed too little information can lead to misunderstanding and even mislead patients. This can be particularly so when discussing diagnosis and prognosis information with the patients and athletes you work with. An easy tip to ensure understanding is to get your patients or athletes to summarise what you have just said.

I routinely get patients and athletes to explain back to me what I have just told them.

I usually say something like…

'When you get home and your [spouse, brother, sister, partner, mate at work…] asks you what the physio said, what will you tell them?'

If they summarise the information well it confirms understanding and I can be happy I have relayed the correct information at the right level.

If they can't summarise the information well, patients may need a little more explanation, and this is an easy and timely place to do it. You don't want to get to session 2 or 3 and have to go back over this information.

You need patients to understand their problems (assessment findings) and the solutions (your treatment plan) with a clear link to how the treatment plan will fix their problems and get them out of pain and back to full health.

This lack of understanding is the primary reason patients start to drop off after two or three sessions as they lack the clarity and understanding of what the plan is.

This can easily be solved by ensuring you deliver information in a way that each individual patient needs and can understand.

Don't Bullshit!

Quite a strong heading but put simply… If you don't know, don't pretend you do.

You will not gain patient trust or buy-in if you bullshit and get things wrong. We all make errors, but don't put yourself in a position to potentially make more.

As you begin to see more complex patients, it can be increasingly more difficult to nail an accurate diagnosis.

Sometimes patients past medical history recall is poor: they forget information or present it inaccurately, which can make your job making sense of this information difficult.

If you are seeing a patient acutely it can often be even more difficult to diagnose an injury.

They may have an unknown mechanism of injury and due to the acute nature of the injury it may be difficult to attain what structures are injured. A combination of pain, swelling and apprehension to testing might make it nearly impossible to distinguish what structures are damaged.

I couldn't tell you the number of times I have been put on the spot to give a diagnosis and prognosis with super acute injuries. This is commonplace in sport as everyone will be asking you for a diagnosis and the likely prognosis including the athlete, their teammates, the head coach, media staff and even fans on your way back to the team bus!

The biggest piece of advice I could give you to avoid making mistakes and putting your neck on the chopping board is don't fall into the trap of trying to please people and give a diagnosis if you can't clearly make one.

I have previously done this; sometimes I was correct with my acute diagnosis, other times I wasn't.

Looking back now, and learning from my own mistakes, I do everything possible to NOT put myself in that position unless I am highly certain of what the acute injury I am assessing is.

Even now, if I am really pushed to make a diagnosis, I don't make one if I have any doubts about what is going on.

I have witnessed extremely experienced and skilled practitioners make big mistakes trying to make hasty diagnoses.

They are acting on emotion, trying to please those pushing for a diagnosis, and not acting on logic.

It is tough; you have that patient in your clinic who has seen several other therapists previously, all of whom have been unable to diagnose and manage their injury successfully and they want YOU to be the therapist that can.

They want an accurate diagnosis, but maybe you can't give it to them at that first consultation.

Maybe it's an athlete who has picked up an injury and has a Cup Final seven days later.

He or she wants a speedy diagnoses given the short turnaround.

They ask you directly 'What is going on and will I play next week?'

These questions are tough to deal with.

Every part of you wants to please your patient or athlete.

This is human nature. It's your emotions overriding your logic as you want to be positive and you want to give them good news.

This is normal – we all want to help our patients and athletes and give them positive news regarding their diagnosis and prognosis.

But we cannot always do that.

I firmly believe it is better to explain that a diagnosis and prognosis cannot be made at that time and that time is necessary to let the injury settle before clear conclusions can be made.

I might say something like…

'There's a few things that could be going on…'

'Your mechanism of injury could fit a few injuries…we want to clear [add injury] and the best way to do this is….'

'Because of the pain and the swelling I'm not able to test you properly; we are better waiting for things to settle a little and then we will have a clearer picture of what is going on.'

In short, if you're not sure, don't pretend you are.

The worst thing you can do is make a rash diagnosis, and be proved wrong when you later reassess, which makes you look and feel inadequate.

Doing this is a one-way ticket to losing the respect and trust of your patients and athletes, and the wider MDT you work with.

Honesty Is Key

Whatever information we deliver we need to be honest with it.

The starting point to any relationship is honesty and if we mislead our patients in any way, they won't trust what we say, and they certainly won't buy in to what we say.

Honesty does work both ways.

You need your patients to be honest with the information they give you i.e. past medical history, to ensure you can do your job effectively and operate competently and have the necessary detail needed to improve their symptoms.

Patients might withhold information and be dishonest with you.

They do this because they don't trust you.

We want to help them and it's so frustrating when we are not given the information we need to help these patients out of pain and back to function.

But if there is no trust between you and your patient, they will not adhere to whatever treatment plan you give them, no matter how good it is.

You need to be honest and transparent with the information you deliver to build a good solid relationship between you and your patient and get the results you both want.

If someone has an eight-week injury, tell them it's an eight-week injury.

Using a mid-grade 2 medial collateral ligament knee injury as an example, I would label that as a six- to eight-week injury, from incidence to return to play.

Some will be back sooner; I've had athletes back playing elite sport at three weeks post-injury, but some make take longer.

This injury could therefore be anything from 3 weeks up to a 12 weeks lay-off.

Evidence and experience indicate six to eight weeks is more likely, so tell your patient or athlete that.

Making promises that you can get them back in four weeks is dumb, as it's unlikely and if unsuccessful it then appears your treatment and rehab plan has failed.

The challenge to then try to get them back on side, after they feel disappointed and frustrated that they are not yet back to full fitness, is very difficult, sometimes even impossible.

Patients will question whether you have what it takes to get them back.

They question you and your treatment plan; some will go and find another therapist.

This is all because you didn't set expectations well and you weren't honest with a realistic time frame.

Patients will often tell you stories of family or friends or something they read off the internet about how long these types of injuries can take. These preconceived ideas and 'knowledge' can be difficult to unpick.

In any setting, patients or athletes that believe they are an 'expert' in their own injury and medical management makes prognosis planning hard, especially so if they had experience of a similar injury before.

Despite these challenges you need to be clear, direct and honest with the information you deliver. Your diagnosis and prognosis must be honest and realistic.

Whilst we are respectful of any patient's injury, we should aim to push all our patients to get them back to their desired hobbies, occupations and sports as soon as possible. But don't make promises you cannot keep.

As we discussed earlier in the chapter, don't make decisions on emotion; rather use your logic.

Patients and members of the MDT will remember what you say and, ultimately, we live and die professionally by what we *say* we can deliver and what we *actually* deliver.

Be mindful if you use time frames, like six to eight weeks; most people will hear the six and not the eight.

Most people will want to put a positive spin on a negative situation (their injury) and will discard the possible longer time frame.

They want to believe they will be back in six weeks and not eight weeks. That increases the pressure on you to get them back quickly.

This is additionally difficult when patients start to think maybe they could knock a week or two off that time frame. So, what started as a possible eight-week injury is now four weeks!

This problem can be avoided if you are transparent, clear and honest with the information you deliver at the very beginning.

Using clear and honest communication will help you build trust with your patients and make them adhere to their treatment plans.

Explain The WHY...

This is most probably the cornerstone to patient adherence to any treatment plan.

You might have designed the best training or rehab plan for your patient, but if the patient doesn't understand the purpose and goals of the plan you may not reach the desired goal.

You need to explain the phase of each intervention, the purpose of that exercise within that session, the session goal and the plan for that week, the next session and beyond.

By explaining the why, you are giving your patient a plan as to how they are going to get from their current position (injured) to their desired outcome (end goal – pain-free and back to their desired hobbies, occupation or sport).

Being able to give a patient clear reasons why you are doing something and how that intervention links to their desired outcome shows patients you have the 'competence' and the 'substance' behind what you are delivering.

This very lack of substance or perceived lack of substance makes patients question what you are doing and question your skills as a therapist.

Clearly getting your patients to buy-in is key to any intervention you make.

If patients don't trust and believe what we are telling them they are less likely to buy-in and thus any planned intervention may fall by the wayside.

Building trust is key to buy-in and will help strengthen the relationship between you and the patients you work with.

As discussed in this chapter this trust and the respect that comes with it, extends past your patients and includes your peers and senior colleagues.

Do you want to be 'protected' by senior staff, only being allowed to treat simple injuries?

Or do you want to be challenged and see more complex patients and pathologies?

Do you want more responsibility within the department you work in and are sick of being seen as a young and inexperienced therapist?

Gaining this trust and respect from both your patients and the senior staff you work with is the only way you will get given more responsibility and the only way you will start to climb the promotion ladder.

These skills can be difficult to learn and master, even more so because they were not even acknowledged during our university training.

Our university studies focused on the clinical skills and didn't give us other important skill-sets, like how to build rapport and communicate effectively to allow us to gain the trust and respect we deserve as qualified therapists.

It is the failure of these non-clinical skill-sets that prevent so many New Grads ever actually achieving their goals and becoming competent, confident and competitive New Grad Physios.

I know from my own experience that unless you learn these skills you will come unstuck, as patients and athletes will not adhere to your treatment plan and in turn their symptoms will not improve.

The ability to apply these non-clinical skills can be the difference between a good and great therapist.

You can have all the knowledge base in the world but if you can't use this knowledge you will always be fighting an uphill battle when trying to get your patients out of pain and back to full fitness.

To become that competent, confident and competitive New Grad Physio you need to gain the trust and respect of both your patients and senior colleagues, and you need the skill-sets to build rapport and effectively communicate your message if you want to get patients to adhere to your treatment plan.

If you are wondering why some of your patients are not adhering to your current treatment plans, even though you know these programmes will get them better, your ability to communicate your message is the reason.

These skills are so important that I have devoted an individual module to each of these topics within the New Grad Physio Membership.

I teach individual modules showing New Grads:

- How To Gain The Trust & Respect You Deserve From Both Your Patients and Senior Colleagues
- How To Build Rapport & Communicate Effectively With Your Patients and Senior Colleagues
- How To Get Your Patients To Adhere To Your Treatment Plans

With these skills, therapists are no longer perceived as lacking authority and are no longer left feeling frustrated, angry and demotivated when their patients don't adhere to their treatment plans.

They have the competency in both their clinical and non-clinical skills to get patients to trust what they are saying and as a result these patients perform every rep of every set prescribed and as a result get better, and quick.

There is so much more than just being a great hands-on therapist and having the ability to write a great treatment programme.

If you can't effectively implement these with your patients, if you can't build rapport and communicate effectively and if you don't build the trust and respect from your patients and senior colleagues then you will never become that competent, confident and competitive New Grad Physio.

For three more ways to get your patients to buy-in to your treatment plans, check out my video completely FREE at **www.newgradphysio.com/resources**

CHAPTER 8
Competency 4 How to get your next promotion

Now that you have started to gain proficiency in your clinical skills you will start to gain the belief you can progress and move up the promotion ladder.

Moving up the promotion ladder is challenging, as a higher role brings even more expectation and responsibility.

But even before that, getting promoted is a big challenge.

This signals a progression from Stage 3 **'Consciously Competent'** to Stage 4 **'Unconsciously Competent'** on the New Grad Physio Competency Ladder.

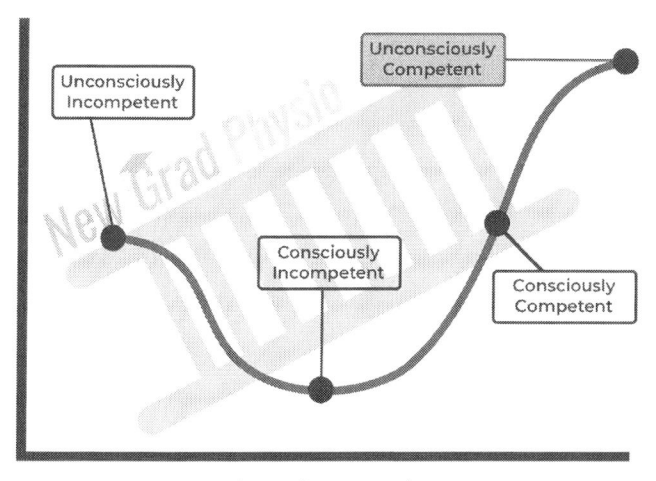

Figure 4 – New Grad Physio Competency Ladder Stage 4. Adapted from (Burch, 1970).

At a clinical level, therapists operating at an Unconsciously Competent level are starting to build towards 'mastery', whereby their clinical skills become second nature.

Therapists at this stage start to 'specialise' in an area, consistently seeing more complex patients and athletes, planning and implementing high level rehab and managing their own caseload efficiently. Additional responsibilities include supporting and mentoring others i.e. junior staff, leading In-Service Training (IST) sessions and giving more input with organisational and managerial tasks.

This would reflect a therapist working at Band 6 level or above in the NHS, an autonomous private practice therapist or a therapist working at first team level within sport.

Whilst these therapists are skilled, they still acknowledge that they need additional support to take the next step in their career. This is usually where you see such therapists pursuing and completing MSc level qualifications and specialist training relative to their current role.

If you have anything about you as a therapist, you will want to pursue your career to the highest level.

Regardless of whether that is in the NHS, private practice or sport, whilst these more senior roles bring about a higher level of responsibility and challenge, the rewards you get and the subsequent job satisfaction are worth it.

But how do you get into a higher position and gain that next promotion?

The content in this chapter will help show you what you need to know, how to make opportunities happen and how to make sure you are ready once those opportunities present themselves.

Lack Of Promotion Skills

Like becoming proficient at your patient assessments, hands-on treatment techniques and rehab implementation, getting promoted is as much about being good at writing a good CV and interviewing well as it is about how good you are clinically.

Progressing to higher roles brings its fair amount of clinical challenges and even therapists operating at this level seek clarity in their patient assessments and management as the complexity of their patient caseload increases.

Being a specialist in one area means that you are meant to be able to fix 'everyone', even those 'tricky' patients other therapists have failed to fix.

But this specialist tag often leaves even senior therapists feeling inadequate and maybe even 'false' in the sense that, even like a New Grad, they question if they are as good as they think they are or as they are perceived to be.

As you move up through the promotion ladder, you become more direct about where you want to end up.

But as you move up the promotion ladder there are increasingly less roles.

This makes the task of getting that interview and getting that job very challenging and is not helped by the fact that at no point in our training, are we ever given any substantial career progression skills.

As mentioned earlier in the book, the best clinical candidates don't always get the best opportunities and jobs.

It's the therapists who can showcase their skills and personality in the best possible way that usually prevail.

This is regardless of the level, whether you are applying for your first job straight from university or applying for a head physiotherapist role at a top sports team.

The job description and requirements will differ, but you need to have the ability to write a knockout CV to get an interview and then possess the skills needed to give a good account of yourself in the interview room.

You can have the best clinical skills in the world but if you are unable to write a great CV and interview well you will never get the opportunity to showcase these skills.

Are You Ready?

We spoke earlier in the book about being CV-ready and how important that is to maximise the chances of getting you that important interview. Regardless of role and the job you are applying for, you will come up short if your CV is poor.

I've screened many CVs and excluded very good candidates because their CV was presented poorly.

It's a formal document and reflects you; more specifically it reflects the level of time and effort you have put in, which may indicate how much you want the role you are applying for.

So, it's a given your CV must be top drawer to give you a chance of getting an interview in the first place.

There are many different roles you might apply for, different departments, NHS versus private practice, different sports teams or organisations etc. and your CV must reflect this.

So many therapists make the mistake of not making their CV specific enough to the area they are applying for. The main reason for this is that many therapists use cookie-cutter templates from the internet to model their CV.

The main issue in doing this is that these CVs are not made by therapists and they don't reflect what is needed in a therapy job application. They are largely built by recruitment companies and job advertising companies and as a result are generic at best. They lack any relevance to the important features that a therapy CV must contain.

If you've previously applied for roles but have been left feeling frustrated, confused, demotivated and feeling 'stuck' that you can't progress, your poor CV writing may be the primary cause.

So, what can you do to write a knockout CV? This topic could be a book in itself given its importance.

To reflect this, I have devoted a full module within the New Grad Physio Membership to CV writing, which includes therapy specific examples, including my own CV I used to gain a role working at an international level in a sport I had no previous experience of working in.

In addition, there is also another module within the membership specifically built to prepare therapists for therapy interviews.

The challenges of firstly getting an interview and then actually nailing that interview and getting that job offer are barriers that so many therapists get stuck at.

That is why I have built these modules to help therapists overcome these challenges and give themselves the best chance of not only progressing up the promotion ladder but progressing up the promotion ladder faster than they ever thought possible.

Showcase Your EGO!

Without coming across as being full of yourself, you need to showcase what you can do and make yourself stand out from the crowd. Too many CVs read the same – a likely result of using those generic internet-ready CV templates.

I have been involved in many interview processes, including CV screening and the interview process itself.

Dependent upon the role, those reading, and screening CVs may have hundreds of applications to work through.

So, to make yours stand out, it needs to be good and it needs to be different.

If I were to put the last ten CVs and letters of application I received side by side, I reckon 75 per cent of the content in each one would be the same.

Whilst an application should have some similarities, as applicants will follow the same job description, the bulk of the content and how this content is displayed should be different.

Remember the job description is what it says. It is detailed information about your roles and responsibilities in the advertised job.

It is not a guide as to what to write in your letter of application.

Attributes like being punctual, having a smart appearance and being enthusiastic are prerequisites; not just for a job as a therapist but for most other professions.

Without these it's unlikely you will succeed in having a long and successful career working in the NHS, private practice or professional sport.

Turning up late will not only lose you the respect of your peers and senior staff, it'll almost always be a one-way ticket to your P45.

So, given these skills are prerequisites, it's unnecessary to include them in your CV.

What readers want to know is something about YOU that makes you different and/or better than the other candidates applying for the same opportunity or job.

Try thinking of something that will grab the reader's attention and is likely to stick in their head.

This not only makes you stand out but also provides a potential topic of conversation, should you make it to the interview stage.

You don't have to have gained 99 A* in your exams or have won an Olympic Gold medal.

You could include interesting places you've seen or interesting things you've done; they don't necessarily need to be specific to the role you are applying for.

They just need to be about you.

The most recent job applications I was involved in, one candidate talked about when he appeared on TV on *Deal Or No Deal,* whilst studying at university, a topic that was brought up at interview.

Talking about these experiences as a candidate is much easier than traditional style interview questions and helps you relax and bring a less formal complexion to the interview.

I've yet to meet any person who enjoys being interviewed; it's a tough and challenging experience for anyone.

So, any help to make it less formal and help you relax can only be a good thing.

So, highlight what is good about YOU.

Don't just quote a generic skill set of qualities that 99 per cent of other applicants will also write. Showcase your EGO and stand out from the crowd. Don't hold back and go hard highlighting your strengths.

We all have something that we are good at, or something good we have achieved or something we are particularly proud of.

Getting this information across is key. It gives an insight into YOU, what you're about, your background and what you've done and achieved.

Make It Professional

Always remember you are applying for a professional job so your CV should reflect this.

Using comical email addresses, nicknames and the like are not appropriate for obvious reasons, but you would be surprised by what aspiring therapists use on their CVs.

Additionally, readers don't need ALL your details. Unless they specifically ask for it, they don't need your full address, NI number, tax code, waist size and inside leg. These are not warranted at this stage.

Your contact details should be easily visible at the top of the page and should include only your name, profession, email and primary telephone number. That is enough information to know who you are and how to contact you if needed. And positioning your details at the top of the page means they can easily be found. The worst thing that could happen is your CV is accepted but the reader struggles to find your contact details and as a result you are not contacted and given an interview. I have seen this happen before.

Using fancy fonts and backgrounds isn't worthwhile for any CV and may in fact detract from the important information that is written on the page itself. Stick with plain text fonts (Times New Roman, Mistral, Calibri or Arial are good choices) and ensure you use the same font throughout the document.

Reading your CV shouldn't read like a story, so be sure to write in the first person. Sentences like 'Andy is… Andy did… Andy has a passion for…' sound like some sort of dramatic play rather than text that should be included as part of your CV.

In addition, only use appropriate and relevant terminology. Using a thesaurus to find flashy wording that no one knows the meaning of may switch off your reader.

Be sure to check spelling, grammar and language. In today's day and age with the use of spellchecker there is really no excuse to be making such errors when writing up your CV. But to double-check, get more than one person to proofread it before sending.

Check, check and double-check your contact details. I know of some applicants that have incorrectly listed their email and phone numbers which in turn resulted in them not being offered an interview, simply because they couldn't be contacted quickly.

Finally, be sure to save and send as a Word document not PDF and make sure you save it with an appropriate name. Remember the person opening your email at the other end will see your file name, so something like 'Physiotherapy Job Application Leeds United' isn't going to look good if you're applying for a physiotherapy role at Leeds Rhinos! If you are applying for more than one role make sure you save a separate file, appropriately named. Note: I have seen this happen before, several times! These people didn't make the interview stage.

Get Your Pitch Right

It has previously been reported that employers look at a CV for an average of 8.8 seconds.

Even the fastest and most efficient readers aren't going to get through much of your CV in that amount of time.

Therefore, you need to grab the reader's attention right at the start of your CV by making the first few sentences engaging so they want to carry on reading.

I call these first few sentences your PITCH.

Like pitching a business idea in the Dragons Den or trying to convince your mates to go on a night out when they really don't want to, it's all about the PITCH and how you SELL your message.

This pitch will be the opening paragraph at the top of your CV and the first thing your reader, your intended employer, will read.

The aim of the PITCH is to engage your reader by showcasing and selling YOUR key skills and attributes. As employers, they want to know what your unique selling points are in relation to the job role being offered.

These might be a specific skill set you have or something you have experienced previously. They could relate to your interests (both career and non-career related), the qualifications you have and/or any other passions you may follow.

Employers want to know what you can bring to the job and be engaged enough by your pitch to want to find out more about you and in turn carry on reading your CV.

As the aim is to grab attention and spark the reader's interest, as a guide, I'd aim to keep your pitch to under eight sentences. If you can't 'pitch' yourself in under eight sentences, then you risk losing the reader's attention and your CV might be one of those read for 8.8 seconds, then tossed by the wayside.

This is without question the hardest section of your CV to write BUT is most definitely the most important part.

Get your pitch right and potential employers will stay engaged and want to continue reading to find out more about you.

Don't Tell Lies

This seems quite an obvious point but you'd be surprised at how many people do tell tales in their desperation to get a job.

Gaining that next promotion is difficult but don't be tempted to mislead your future employer as this may have the opposite effect.

For any medical department, regardless if that is in the NHS, private practice or sport, you don't have to go too far to know someone that knows someone, and so on.

As a result, it's not hard to gain information about a possible future employee should that be necessary.

Previously in the book I spoke about how you can use 'research' to find out about those you are contacting to maximise the chances of you making opportunities for yourself.

In the same way, employers will do their own 'research' on potential candidates.

Why wouldn't they?

If they can find out about what a potential candidate is really like, how they communicate with patients and staff, their ability as a therapist, they will do it.

Some people can look great on paper (CV) and talk the talk in their interview but are not the real deal when they start working.

This process of research takes this element of risk out of the equation.

I have selected, and deselected, therapists for interview after having spoken to other professionals who have worked with these individuals previously.

So, if you choose to make information up or mislead employers with what you are saying you might be shooting yourself in the foot.

If you say you have 'worked' somewhere, make sure you have. This is a big error made by both students and New Grads, whereby they mislead and imply they have worked somewhere previously when they haven't. 'Working' somewhere implies a paid position where you have received income for your services. Shadowing or completing a formal or informal placement is therefore not work.

Several times I have spoken to other professionals working at other clubs where applicants have claimed they have 'worked' at that club; however, they never have. Equally other professionals have contacted me asking about interview candidates who claimed they had 'worked' alongside me; however, they never had.

None of these people got an interview.

Just recently a former student who had completed a placement with me put me down as a reference for a job application.

She made two big errors.

Firstly, she didn't tell me I was a reference. Whilst I would never mind being a reference for anyone, it is courteous to ask people before you do.

Secondly, she stated in her application that she had worked at the professional sports club I was working at, when she had in fact only completed a placement. Her potential employer contacted me directly for clarification on this. I was honest with the information I gave, and she didn't get an interview.

She's probably unaware of why she didn't get an interview and is possibly still making the same mistake over and over, not getting interviews and probably wondering why.

Whilst examples like these are fortunately rare, they highlight an important issue.

Don't try to mislead. Be transparent with what you say and the information you deliver to prospective employers.

Transparency goes above and beyond applying for jobs.

Earlier in the book I discussed how important it is to gain the trust from your patients and colleagues if you want to be a successful New Grad Physio. Transparency underpins everything we do when working as a therapist.

You will not gain the trust of your peers, your patients and the senior colleagues you work with without transparency.

Being competent at what you do will instigate trust, but without transparency that trust will not last.

Don't lie or mislead potential employers as it might come back to bite you.

How To Smash Your Interview

What should you expect in an interview?

What is the expected format and content?

What will you be asked and what will you be made to do?

Whilst there will always be some degree of the unknown to any interview, you can prepare yourself well so you are ready to take on the challenge and give the best account of yourself possible.

I've had the pleasure of being the right side of the desk on many occasions, interviewing others, and fortunately not had the displeasure too many times of being interviewed myself.

You see, I have used many of the skills I am presenting in this book and the many more I teach in the New Grad Physio Membership to skip the interview process and gain a promotion.

If you do your job right and know what to do, what to say and how to say it, you may also be able to do this.

That said, most therapists will go through the traditional model of promotion, including a face-to-face interview.

The interview process is often the number one aspect aspiring New Grads fear the most. But if you are well prepared it doesn't have to be.

Any therapy interview will broadly follow the same format and content.

- General human resources questioning
- Questioning to gain more knowledge about you
- Case study or scenario-based questions

There are many questions you are likely to be asked, many of which you can practice your response to.

The biggest question you must ask yourself is WHY are they asking ME this question?

If you can get in the head of the interviewer, you will have a good idea the type of answer they are looking for.

Whilst there will never be a PERFECT answer there is always a WRONG one!

Regarding the human resource questions, it is important to do your research regarding the organisation you are intending to work for.

This might include what is current in that hospital, clinic or sports club.

If you falter on this part of the interview, answering basic questions about the organisation you are intending to work for, it won't get you off to the best start.

This bit is easy as all the current updates and news will likely be presented on the organisation's website.

The second section of the interview is designed to give the interviewers the opportunity to gain more knowledge about you.

You might get asked questions like:

- *Why did you apply for the role and what skills and attributes can you bring to it?*
- *Can you give us an example of a mistake that upon reflection you might have done differently at the time?*
- *Can you tell us about your experience with [insert: treatment technique, rehab, programming]?*
- *Can you give us an example of a success story with a player/patient you have worked with in the past?*
- *What difficulties do you think you may encounter with this role?*
- *What are your selling points?*

These are questions used to clarify any questions and reservations your potential employers might have about you based on your application but are also a BIG opportunity for you to sell yourself and showcase why they should give you the job.

The questions ask you to reflect on both your successes and mistakes, and are asking you what you have learned and how you have improved your practice following these previous experiences.

Questions about your experiences with specific treatment techniques, rehab or programming are trying to distinguish if your current skill-sets align with the skills needed to work in the environment and role you are applying for.

Finally, most interviews close with some sort of case study or scenario-based questions.

These could be just questions but could also be role plays or practical based tasks that will require a differing level of response and action.

You should have an idea what is to be expected in this section as your interview details should indicate this.

Case studies or scenarios usually include one or more of the following:

- Injury, Programming or Coaching Example(s)
- Conflict-Resolution Scenario(s)

These are used to give the employer an idea of your current level, both your knowledge and the application (or proposed application) of your knowledge.

The conflict-resolution scenarios are commonly used because they are real.

Working in any medical department there will always be differing opinions of how patients or athletes should be managed. Differing members of the MDT will have different ideas and this will undoubtedly result in conflict.

The ability to deal with conflict and being able to reason your own argument and opinions is a key skill any therapist needs, particularly so the more senior the role you hold.

It's probably not even a skill, rather an ART. And it is this ART of collaboration that is often the big difference between successful therapists and unsuccessful therapists.

Working within any medical department, NHS, private practice or professional sport, a key to success is being able to communicate and interact well with other people.

The best relationships and the best teams are usually not the product of the best individuals but of individuals that work very well together.

This is true whether we are relating this to a busy NHS department, a private practice clinic or a professional sports team, or any other industry for that matter.

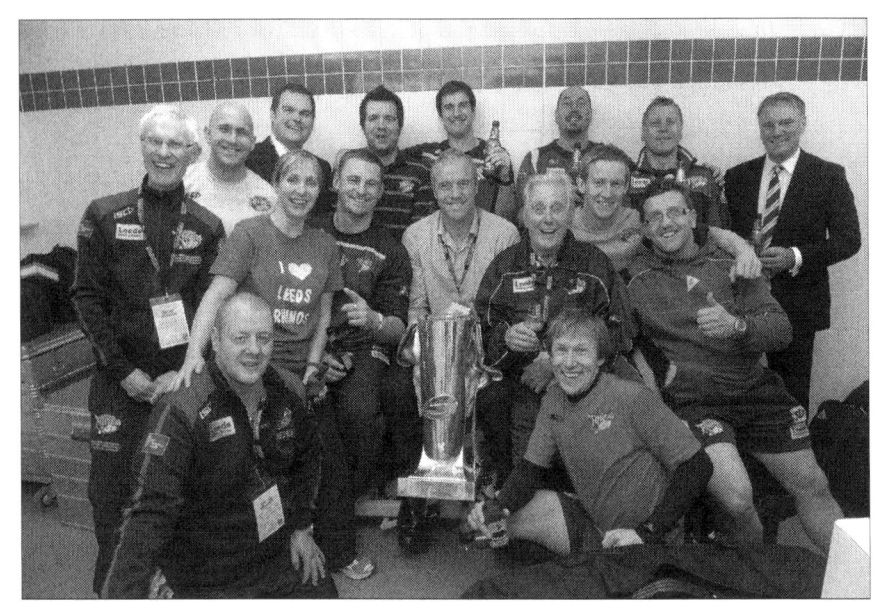

The backroom staff enjoying a beer after a Grand Final Win with the Leeds Rhinos

As a physiotherapist, I have my own thoughts and opinions about other areas that I am not directly involved in.

In sport, this would include my opinion on the coaching, strength and conditioning, sports science and nutrition practices employed. Equally, these professionals will have an opinion on my physiotherapy practices and the medical department, and rightly so.

Having worked with a variety of different departments with many different professionals for many years, one of the major lessons that I have learnt is that the ability to collaborate is key to the success of any team.

The ability to collaborate is not something that was taught during our studies, whether we are healthcare professionals, strength and conditioning coaches, skills coaches, nutritionists or any other type of professional.

I remember being told about the MDT and how important it is for different professionals to work well together to achieve a common goal. And whilst this is true, nobody ever talked about how to do this and why or how an effective MDT operates.

My first big piece of advice about how to collaborate well in any MDT is to **Not Avoid Conflict.**

There will always be times when you might have a differing opinion to others. I often do, as I'm sure you do, and sometimes these opinions need to be voiced.

But before you jump straight in there and throw yourself in at the deep end, you may want to ask for clarity regarding a discussion point.

A clinical decision might have been made considering some information that you are not aware of. Asking for clarity as to why that decision was made will give you the information you need to understand the reasons behind it.

Jumping the gun and trying to make an argument without all the information is a quick-fire way of getting someone's back up and is unlikely to result in a successful outcome.

If you know and understand why that decision has been made, then that initial difference of opinion is no longer an issue. Had you jumped straight down somebody's throat questioning everything under the sun unnecessarily, it's likely this would have caused conflict and a subsequent possible heated discussion.

Continued conflict within any medical department is something we obviously want to avoid where possible.

There are times, however, where you need to voice your opinion even if it is in direct opposition to another member of the team. If it needs to be said then you need to say it.

Maybe even after asking for clarification and following the steps discussed above, the answers you receive might not sit well with you.

In these cases, you must speak up. If you think these decisions are going to be of detriment to a patient or athlete under your care, in any way, you must voice your opinion, even if this is outside your field of expertise.

Of primary importance is the patient or athlete we are working with and if something needs to be said, say it.

But how do you voice your concerns and opinions?

This is hard, particularly so if you lack perceived experience and knowledge around more senior therapists and other members of the MDT.

To do this, firstly, you must be strong in your judgement and be sure you have some substance behind your opinion. This more relates to your clinical skills and having a clear understanding and clarity regarding your patient assessments and interventions.

You need to be clear about what you are saying and have the substance to validate your claim(s) and in turn make your argument a strong one.

Secondly, you need to be sure to consider your surroundings.

Certain personalities can become very defensive if questioned. Therefore, bringing up your potential issue might not be best suited within a departmental meeting in front of a larger group.

If possible, it may be more appropriate to speak to individuals like this in close quarters away from the group. If you know there might be a possible conflict and what you say could be taken the wrong way, a process like this could help to minimise a potential confrontation and ultimately your message and resultant recommendation(s) are more likely to be acted upon.

Equally, it is sometimes of value speaking to other members of the MDT beforehand to tee them up about possible discussion points, as their opinions and support in the meeting may help your cause.

As you build a relationship and rapport with those you work with, you will ascertain how they work and, more importantly, how they like to receive information.

This information is key to then allow you to structure your message in the correct way.

Is one person right and another wrong? Probably not. They are probably just looking at the same issue from a different perspective.

To further enhance collaboration, I have learnt over many years that you need to be both a good giver and a good receiver of information.

Despite sometimes having differing opinions from other members of the MDT, you can still get to the same common goal for your patients and athletes by collaborating well. The ability to do this quite often yields faster and better patient results.

One member of the MDT might be more dominant during a certain period i.e. a surgeon during the operating decision-making process or a therapist during the rehab phase but input from all the MDT is always warranted and needed.

Above all, the ability to collaborate is key. Many different disciplines will have differing opinions on a variety of different topics. Whatever these opinions, the common goal is always the same: to improve patient symptoms and get them back to full fitness.

How we get to that point may be open to opinion but what is clear is that collaborating as a team will allow all disciplines their input and if these inputs don't conflict with one another we should be able to work towards this common goal.

What Makes A Good Team Player?

A good team player is most often a GIVER and a TAKER. So, which one are you?

Are you the one that always helps others out, like your colleagues at work, or are you the one that takes what you can from all of those around you to maximise personal gain?

Some of us will probably lean towards one side or the other and this may change as we move up the promotion ladder and our roles and responsibilities change.

I guess you would like to think you are more of a giver than a taker, but are you?

Within the business world, recent evidence has suggested that although takers tend to be more successful financially the givers are generally in a better position to advance their careers and sustain greater longevity once they reach the top of their field.

So, within the business world if you're after a quick buck, take from those around you, get them to do the hard yards and you'll reap the benefits, at least in the short-term.

But if you're after long-lasting success and longevity you are better being a giver. You might not reap the benefits as quickly, but you should expect a longer and more sustainable stay at the top once you get there.

Although this relates to the business world, there is big carry-over into your role as a therapist.

I have spoken at length about the importance of building relationships, both with your patients and the MDT to ensure a successful working environment and positive patient outcomes. We know that a poor relationship between you and your patient will likely lead to poor treatment, rehab and performance outcomes. The flip side is that a strong relationship should lead to good treatment, rehab and positive patient outcomes.

As therapists we tend to have closer and stronger relationships with the patients we work with, much closer than other members of the MDT are often able to make.

I believe there are two main reasons for this.

Firstly, time. As therapists we are a big part, the main part, of any recovery and rehab process, which for many patients presents the bulk of their care.

The larger amount of time we spend with our patients gives us a bigger opportunity to build these positive relationships, assuming we know how to build rapport and patient trust.

Secondly, I believe that patients think we have their best interests at heart.

When we are assessing, treating and rehabilitating our patients we devise a plan based on the best interests of that patient at that time.

This is a strong example of being a 'giver'. When patients see this behaviour consistently, they put trust in us and we can build a stronger relationship, largely because they appreciate our 'giving' approach.

Should they think we are driven by other things or have different motives, aside from their best interests, then they don't trust or buy into what we do and say.

As a result, this important patient–therapist relationship is much weaker and, in turn, we can expect higher levels of patient non-adherence to rehab, and poor clinical and patient outcomes.

This giver-taker relationship gets a little more complex when we start to consider the context of the situation, the person(s) receiving the information and the intended outcome expected.

At times we might be more of a giver or more of a taker and this will be directly relevant to the situation presenting.

If you don't feel that you fit into either category i.e. you're neither predominately a giver or a taker, maybe you are not. You could be a MATCHER.

Givers generally find out ways to be helpful and give to others. Takers focus on extracting as much as possible from others. Matchers play 'tit for tat' – they reciprocate and expect reciprocity and, as such, fall somewhere between the two.

But as discussed, there are situations when we act differently and everyone – even givers – can operate like takers.

Despite these situational changes I believe that we all have a dominant type i.e. we are predominately a giver, a taker or a matcher. We can change and adapt. Our goals and motives will be the primary drive behind which style we predominately adopt.

Previous academic work suggests that givers and matchers run the risk of becoming takers when they disregard their actions and the consequence these actions have on other people.

In life we often feel the need to pigeonhole ourselves into one category or another.

Are you a giver, taker or matcher?

Does it really matter?

All we do know is that people will generally adopt one style more than another. The important factor is highlighting the drive behind which style they choose to adopt. The goals and motives of someone will likely be the deciding factor as to which style is most dominant.

Can we change? Sure, we can change our style, but such changes are the likely consequence of a change in motive.

What is clear however in a therapy domain is the need to be adaptable and at times we will need to take the position of a taker, a giver or even a matcher.

This is a key component in the art of collaboration and key to any successful MDT.

How To Fast-Track Your Career

As you are probably starting to realise, the ability to climb up the promotion ladder relies on your abilities both clinically and non-clinically.

Non-clinically, these skills include the ability to write a knockout CV and smash your interview, giving you the best chance to fast-track your career.

These skills are learnt processes, and you can become much better at these skills very quickly. Problem is, nobody has ever taught us these skills.

Having worked with so many New Grad Physios I know the current challenges you are facing and as such I have created a support programme, the New Grad Physio Membership, to help you learn these skills.

I have dedicated modules to help you develop both your clinical skills and non-clinical skills, like CV writing and interview preparation, as I know these can be the main factor helping you to get a job or that next promotion.

If you have struggled in the past trying to get an interview, or indeed got an interview but didn't get offered a job, you may have made some of the mistakes presented in this chapter.

What did you do after you received these negative responses?

Did you just accept the decision; maybe blame something or someone else?

Did you contact the employer to ask for feedback?

What is always worth considering is that there might have been someone better at that time, a candidate who performed better than you both on paper and at the interview.

There might have been an internal promotion and the employers might have already had a favourite candidate in mind prior to the interview process.

If you are unsuccessful it is always worthwhile asking for feedback. The information provided might help you in future applications and highlight some of the mistakes you may have made with your application.

It can be hard reaching out and knowing what to say to get constructive feedback that you can turn into positives following disappointing news.

Therefore, I have produced a resource you can use to send to employers if you have been unsuccessful at either the CV stage or the interview stage itself.

You can get it here for FREE at www.newgradphysio.com/resources

What is also important to remember is that you should never burn bridges if you are unsuccessful; reaching out to employers even if you don't make the grade can be beneficial.

It not only gives you the opportunity to gain important feedback it also gives you the opportunity to express your interest in other opportunities that might be available or might come up soon.

Progressing up the promotion ladder is as hard as you make it.

You need to act to be the best prepared you can be to make the most of your opportunities when they arise.

The ability to write a knockout CV and the ability to smash your interview are two big challenges that all New Grad Physios face, in addition to the many clinical challenges.

Similarly, both these clinical and non-clinical skills need practice and you need to get better at them if you wish to become that competent, confident and competitive New Grad Physio and progress up the promotion ladder.

As you progress in your career, further challenges and problems that you will need to navigate will present themselves.

As additional content within the New Grad Physio Membership, I teach members how to negotiate contract terms of employment, how to secure additional 'bonuses' or 'allowances' for CPD or ongoing training and even how to amend certain roles, to allow changes in responsibility and allow reduction in working hours and/or increases in salary.

This ability to negotiate salary and contract terms can be the difference in £1000s in money in your pocket and the opportunity to advance your skills further with additional training and CPD paid for by your employer.

It is the same know-how I used myself to get my Master's degree fully paid by my employer and to negotiate with the university to let me take the degree part-time.

This made the degree achievable to complete alongside working full-time, and saved me over £6000 in tuition fees.

There are many challenges you will face trying to progress your career and go up the promotion ladder, but there's so much you can do to make this process much smoother.

To find out more about how to act and start moving up the promotion ladder faster than you ever thought possible, visit **www.newgradphysio.com**

CHAPTER 9
How to hit the ground running in the NHS as a New Grad Physio

Working in different areas presents different obstacles and working in the NHS brings its own unique challenges.

In relation to physiotherapy, your previous studies are more closely aligned to this environment, with teachings driven in most cases by current and previous NHS staff, and the content driven towards NHS provision.

Other therapy degrees, like sports therapy and sports rehabilitation, follow different learning content; however, more roles for non-physiotherapist positions within the NHS are becoming more common, so the content in this chapter applies to all therapy professions.

Furthermore, the content of physiotherapy course programmes has started to change in recent years and is likely to continue to do so moving forwards.

Previously all physiotherapy degrees, both BSc and MSc programmes, were funded by the NHS so, as a student, you didn't pay any tuition fees. This funding provision has now been stopped, and the cost per year of tuition fees has risen sharply in recent years.

Now that NHS funding has been removed, universities are seemingly taking more control of their own course programmes, which can only be a good thing moving forwards. Such changes will allow institutions to alter the curriculum, update content and deliver more of what is needed to equip New Grad Physios for the real world.

However, such changes are likely to take time.

One of the biggest frustrations New Grads speak to me about is that university teachings are rigid and too generalised. They feel that although they cover a very broad spectrum of areas, which is needed, they don't go into enough depth in any one area.

This leaves New Grad Physios feeling underprepared for when they do start to work in the NHS as a Band 5 therapist.

Furthermore, whilst duration of rotations will vary from trust to trust, many therapists feel because they are frequently moving from one area to another, they de-skill as they are not using certain skills day-to-day.

For example, as a New Grad you may start with a respiratory rotation, then after 3–4 months you may rotate to neurology, to MSK, to orthopaedics or another area.

Therapists often tell me they feel they are just getting into their stride before they are asked to move to another area.

Assessments and interventions will differ from one specialist area to another so therapists are continually having to relearn new assessment formats, protocols and treatment techniques that are unique to each area.

This continual change can lead to frustration and the reality of NHS rotations is that you will rotate to some areas that you don't have a big interest in. This is hard, having to work in an area that you don't have a passion for and an area you don't see yourself working in, in the long-term.

You feel like you are wasting your time, and your time would be much better spent working in the area you know you want to pursue longer term.

You may, for example, want to work in MSK Outpatients, but you are continually unsuccessful every time you request this rotation.

MSK rotations particularly are very popular and in short supply and can therefore cause major frustration for many New Grad Physios.

This is a direct question I got asked recently by a Band 5 New Grad Physio:

'I'm currently waiting to get into my MSK rotation as I didn't get one as a student and I feel I lack the basic assessment skills gained from seeing patients regularly in that environment.

I have done a lot of volunteering at events and I help at a local rugby club but when I try to shadow the physio on a training night, it is often very quiet and hard to get exposure.

Even when I do see patients, I'm not able to take those skills away and practice as I don't have the regular patients to practice on.

I'm hugely lacking experience and confidence in my MSK assessment skills and I'm wondering if there's anything I can do to improve these skills whilst waiting for my rotation?' PT (Band 5 NHS Physio)

Having spoken to PT he was becoming increasingly frustrated by his lack of opportunities. He was very clear that he wanted to pursue a career in the NHS, and MSK is his preferred speciality. Yet he was questioning when this opportunity would happen; how long would he be waiting for that MSK rotation?

He was already close to a year post-graduation and hadn't been able to secure that MSK placement.

He felt he was deskilling daily and this was compounded by the fact that he had gained little MSK experience as a student.

He felt the more and more rotations he did in non-MSK areas, the further away he got from his dream job and the more he was deskilling.

This was causing him to feel demotivated and frustrated, and he was starting to not enjoy going to work.

He was questioning his future career direction and was even considering whether he would have to leave the NHS and pursue a role in private practice, given the lack of opportunities – something that he really didn't want to do.

This is a common problem amongst so many New Grad Physios working within the NHS.

So, what you do if you find yourself in a similar position?

There are steps you can take to gain your desired rotation and stop leaving the decision completely out of your hands.

Gaining YOUR Desired New Grad NHS Rotation

To gain your desired rotation in the NHS you have one of two options:

1 Bide your time and wait

2 Take action

Taking action means actively engaging to make yourself more employable and a New Grad that senior staff want on their next rotation.

The themes we will discuss now can be applied to any area of physiotherapy within the NHS, not just MSK.

If you are happy just waiting, deskilling and becoming more and more frustrated, then keep going with that plan.

But if you want to maximise your chances of being chosen on the next round of rotations, your desired rotation, then you need to know this:

'The best candidates DON'T always get the best roles'.

You could be the best candidate for the next round of rotations, you might really excel in that environment, bring enthusiasm to the post and be a successful addition to the department, but that doesn't mean that you will get the role.

At the end of the day you're most likely just a name on a sheet, competing against many other New Grad Physios for the same rotation.

So how can you make yourself stand out from all the other therapists?

Engage With The Right Department

Whilst you may not be directly working with other therapists, there is no reason why you cannot engage and interact with them.

Firstly, you could try to speak to junior and senior therapists within your desired department. Speak to them and pick their brains to find out what is current in that area; these could be new procedures or protocols they are adhering to or research that they may be involved with.

You could ask senior staff for guidance as to what you could be doing right now to improve your chances of making the cut when they decide the provision for the next round of rotations.

Even just making your intentions clear to a senior member of staff shows drive, shows desire and it shows you genuinely actually want to work in their department.

You get your name and face known so when the next rotations are decided, there is more substance to your name, and you increase the likelihood of a positive outcome.

Furthermore, you could take this a step further.

Is it possible you could attend any CPD or IST sessions?

This is a great way to interact with other therapists, pick up more information relative to that department and at the same time improve your knowledge base.

You might need to make the hours up somewhere else in your working week to facilitate this, but it will be well worth the effort.

If you can't schedule the time to make these CPD sessions, why not consider taking a day's holiday?

If you really want the role, going over and above like this is only going to be seen in a good light and could put you well in front of your peers competing for the same roles.

Make Other Opportunities For Yourself

If you are not currently getting the experience you need, then it is worth considering getting such experience elsewhere.

Whilst you continue to pursue your chosen area, gaining exposure in semi-professional, part-time or amateur sport is a great way to get experience.

For a very small amount of time commitment you can attain REAL hands-on experience and practice your assessment, treatment and rehab skills.

Despite being 'stuck' on a rotation that isn't your thing, you can use your time wisely. You can gain access to an environment that gives you frequent exposure to practice and opportunity to develop your skills set.

PT, the student I detailed above, was doing this. Whilst pursuing his MSK rotation he was helping at a local rugby club, giving him exposure to MSK injuries and their management.

One of the things we discussed was engaging in more opportunities and maybe finding another team or environment whereby he would gain more exposure and more hands-on practice.

Whilst PT had acted and taken steps to secure this rugby exposure, some training nights were quiet and he would have a limited caseload to see, and some match days were low-key, which meant at times he felt like a glorified first-aider, not a qualified physiotherapist.

So, we spoke about exploring other opportunities to maximise his time and spend it wisely. If you are going to take an opportunity like PT did, make sure you are getting out of it what you intend.

There are many roles in semi-professional, part-time and amateur sports that are crying out for New Grad Physios just like you ready to test themselves and maybe even earn some extra cash.

There are further opportunities outside the public sector in other areas of therapy that you could explore. Some shadowing work in a private practice, on an evening or even weekend, might be just what you need to help ensure you are upskilled and ready to make the most of your rotation opportunity when it arises.

Think Like A Band 6

The best way to excel as a band 5 therapist is to model yourself on a band 6 therapist.

Once you've nailed it and have got that 3- or 4-month rotation in the area you see yourself working long term, you want to hit the ground running.

You have a short window to impress senior staff to put yourself in contention for a static role; whether this is a band 5 or even band 6 role.

Even if you're only a band 5, senior staff are looking for attributes in you that would fit a band 6 role. In any environment, including private practice and sport, senior staff are always looking for people that they think will be worth their investment of time, resources and efforts to upskill them with a view to them staying in that environment for the long term.

Nobody is going to put the time and effort into any therapist if they perceive them to only want to be around short-term, before heading off somewhere else.

Senior staff will put their efforts in helping junior therapists **IF** they feel they will progress and have the attributes to make a successful band 6.

So, you need to make it clear to senior staff that you are that person, that you will be that successful band 6, and to do that you therefore need to start thinking like a band 6 therapist.

Firstly, you need to identify what a band 6 in your department does.

Sounds simple, but unless you know what responsibilities a band 6 physio has, then you are just guessing the skills and attributes you need to develop yourself. Knowing exactly what these roles and responsibilities are will help direct your own learning and allow you to be specific to what skills and attributes you prioritise developing.

Many of the band 5 physios that I have coached feel like they lack the rehab skills needed to fully support more active and athletic populations that they might see.

They often feel that interventions like the 'ACL classes' are not enough for some patients but lack the skill-sets to actually prescribe anything different.

They feel they need the exposure to rehab and to learn how to programme higher level exercise to ensure they have the confidence to treat these populations.

And this is not just band 5 therapists.

I have provided teaching to senior staff within NHS Teaching Hospital Trusts with both upper and lower limb rehab courses.

This was delivered to band 6, 7 and 8 MSK staff and was organised because they also felt that they struggled with more athletic populations and wanted to upskill their exercise catalogue, gain a deeper understanding of what high level rehab included and how to reason the inclusion of such rehab for more athletic patients.

Some of these staff were very experienced and had been 'specialising' in MSK for many years.

Due to a combination of lack of exposure, lack of training and lack of resources (equipment and time), they felt they were under-providing a service to their patients, hence the need to organise some training.

As a group they felt they were just giving patients the same exercises time after time and were reluctant to give higher level rehab exercises in fear of causing injury and regression of symptoms.

So, it's not just junior therapists that question their skills and applications.

With that in mind, rehab exercise planning and the application of rehab is something as a band 5 you need to get better at.

A band 5 physio, currently a member of the New Grad Physio Membership, has done just that.

After a coaching call together, she explained many of the issues already discussed above in relation to the struggles of a New Grad working in the

NHS. When we spoke, she was on her MSK rotation but wasn't happy with the rehab provision many of her patients were getting. She questioned the set 'protocols' and 'exercise sheets' that she was being suggested to give out to patients and felt she was selling her patients short.

On the coaching call we discussed a few options and came up with a strategy to overcome this. She then started a small project to redesign the department's ACL pathway. She enlisted the help of a couple of other band 5 therapists to help her and used one of the IST slots to collect ideas from the wider MSK team. As a result, in a short amount of time, she was able to devise a new and updated ACL pathway for the department.

At the time of writing this has been implemented with great success within the department and is being considered for widespread expansion within the full hospital trust! This is a massive achievement, and she feels this was also the primary driver to her recently being offered a static band 6 role, something she gladly accepted.

She felt the project and its implementation put her on the radar of senior staff in the department including consultants and other senior MDT members, who were interested in the project. She was operating at a level higher than her paygrade as a band 5, acting and taking on more responsibility which in turn put her in the driving seat for her promotion.

Band 6 positions require you to take more responsibility. This is a clear example whereby a therapist did exactly that; she was proactive, led other people, conducted some research, presented ideas to the group and was able to affect positive change.

These are the attributes senior staff want and therefore it is no surprise to me that she was offered a promotion soon after this project.

Maybe developing a programme like this might feel like too big a task for you right now. But you could just start with making a conscious effort to get more involved in IST sessions, maybe even take the lead or co-lead a session with another therapist.

Given you will know the topic for discussion beforehand, set some time aside to research the topic area and read some relevant journals so you are prepped and ready to input into the group discussions. If you find a good journal article you could even forward it via email to other staff prior to the training session. This shows foresight and engagement on your part, which will only be seen positively by the rest of the group.

The higher you progress in the NHS system, the more complex and challenging the patients you see will be. It goes without saying that the caseload of a band 5 therapist is very different to that of a therapist operating at band 7 or 8, like an Extended Scope Practitioner.

As a band 5, your first goal must be to become competent and confident treating your own caseload. We have talked about the different levels of competency and the four stages of the New Grad Physio Competency Ladder.

Regardless of whether you work in the NHS, private practice or sport, building competency is key. Only when you are competent and have the confidence in what you are delivering as a New Grad Physio are you ready to progress.

Having built this competency and confidence you will be ready for more complex patients and you will be ready to take on the challenges in your chosen NHS field and to step up to the next level as a band 6 physio.

As a junior therapist you might not get the exposure to some pathologies and injuries. This can be hospital or even trust dependant as many departments will have a screening protocol that filters patients depending upon their referral information i.e. more basic patients are given to band 5 staff and more complex patients to band 6 and band 7 staff.

But there will always be the odd complex patients who slip the net and you might be presented with more complex and difficult cases even as a band 5.

Rather than being daunting, these are great opportunities to showcase how good a therapist you are and that you are worthy and ready for the next step, the next promotion, the next role as a band 6 therapist.

Wouldn't it be great if you had the competence and confidence to treat more complex patients?

What would it be like if you had the confidence in your assessment skills and clarity in your findings to use the correct hands-on treatment techniques, and could implement the correct rehab exercises for each patient that walked through your door?

MSK therapy is an area that is constantly evolving and that is why many NHS New Grad Physios feel they are falling behind and that they are losing track about what is current in this field.

This lack of confidence often means they are reluctant to treat even their own peers, family and friends and they second-guess themselves and question whether they have the skills to find an accurate diagnosis and to implement an effective treatment plan.

Whilst there are many obstacles as a New Grad Physio, some that are specific to working in the NHS, by acting you can create your own opportunities and put yourself in the driving seat once these opportunities present themselves.

Many New Grad Physios are sick of just going through the motions, feeling frustrated on rotations they don't really want, and stagnating in their learning and career progression.

Many New Grad Physios talk to me about their lack of support and the quality of support that they have access to as being a major variable in their lack of progress, both clinically and on the promotion ladder.

Any New Grad Physio can take the necessary steps to move towards their dream role, regardless of the barriers they think are stopping them, but they just need the right support.

CHAPTER 10
How to overcome the challenges of a New Grad Physio working in private practice

Despite having a free socialist healthcare system, there has been a big growth in recent years of patients opting to self-pay, either directly or via private healthcare insurance, for their own therapy.

Patients do this for many reasons including having the flexibility to book appointments at convenient times and at convenient locations around their other commitments, to access longer appointment slots and to self-book and not need a GP referral or need to be put on a waiting list to be seen.

As a therapist, operating in this area brings its own specific challenges.

Given the cost implications on the part of the patient there is without question a larger expectation to get these patients better and quick.

They are choosing to pay for their own care and not to access the NHS; rightly or wrongly they often expect a level of care that reflects this.

As a New Grad Physio working in this area it is likely you are working for someone else in a clinic, but, even then, there is pressure from those senior staff to provide a high level of service.

Being a private practice owner myself, I know that the quality of care the therapists at my clinic deliver are a reflection on me and my business.

If that care falls below patient expectations, then there's a problem.

Patients firstly won't get better and secondly won't come back.

I need to provide a service that gets patients out of pain and back to full fitness and my therapists need to be able to build trust with their patients, so they adhere to their treatment plans, not only so they get better but also so they complete a full package of care.

Any good private practice is built on a good word-of-mouth referral system – patients having a successful recovery from their own injury recommending the clinic to their family and friends.

Yes, a good marketing system and profile on the internet and social media platforms will help attract new patients and engage previous patients but in terms of patient numbers through the door a good word-of-mouth system can't be beaten.

It will ensure a steady stream of new leads and costs the clinic absolutely nothing in marketing.

The big problem in private practice and getting consistent numbers on your caseload is patient drop-off. You see this usually after two to three sessions whereby patients often feel much better, their pain is reduced, maybe even gone altogether, and they don't come back.

They don't see the value in having any additional sessions but as therapists we know they need additional input to complete their care package and ensure when they do return to their chosen activities, their symptoms do not return.

You see, often the easiest part of a patient's treatment plan is taking away their pain. The hardest part is knowing how to keep progressing them, and giving them exposure to the movements and loads they require to ensure they are ready to return to their desired activities, whilst giving the body time to adapt to this graded exposure.

The failure to complete a graded exposure and complete a full treatment plan is why a patient's symptoms quickly return and why they either reinjure or pick up a new injury very soon after they have left your clinic.

Largely speaking, these patients are the ones who have self-discharged and dropped off after a few sessions.

You might be thinking why does this matter? It's not your business, you still get paid the same, there still seems to be a steady stream of patients coming through your clinic door.

But this patient drop-off is a direct reflection of you as a therapist.

If your patients don't complete your proposed plan of care, it's because they haven't seen the value in what you were proposing and/or don't believe and trust in what you are saying.

We spoke about this at length earlier in the book and this is likely down to one of two factors.

You either haven't communicated your treatment plan to your patient well.

Or you don't know how to plan an effective treatment plan, from start to finish, for the patient.

For most New Grad Physios, it's usually a combination of the two, but regardless, if you can't plan out and communicate a treatment plan to your patients, then patient drop-off will continue, and patients will regress. This will be a direct reflection of you and your abilities as a therapist.

You are also doing your patients a disservice, as many of these patients are regressing, their symptoms are returning, and they are right back where they started before they came to see you in the first place.

In the eyes of your private practice boss this isn't good either.

If patients are dropping off and those patients who regress are not referring their friends and family, clinic numbers will drop off and that's a problem for any therapy business.

Business aside, as therapists we want to get our patients better, regardless of whether we work in private practice, the NHS or sport.

If we are unable to take patients through a full treatment plan, we are not giving them the input they need to make a successful return to their desired outcome, and without fear of their symptoms returning.

Being able to take a patient through a full treatment plan will allow you to best serve your patients and at the same time be the star employee, and the therapist who continually gets new word-of-mouth referrals and is seen as that go-to therapist within your clinic.

Patients Are Paying So They Deserve More Time

This is a big misconception New Grads working in private practice make.

Yes, patients are paying with their hard-earned cash and they expect a certain level of service and resources but more time is not what's needed.

Patients want to get better. They want you to take their pain away and get them back to their desired outcome as soon as possible.

Whether their desired outcome is playing sport, gardening or playing with their grandkids, doesn't matter; what they want is results, not more of your time.

A big mistake New Grad Physios make working in private practice is giving patients longer treatment slots.

Maybe you have a gap between patients, so you let a session run over, assuming you are going over and above for your patient. But if you're not getting them better you are doing them a disservice, regardless of how long you make their appointment slot.

The pressure is especially big in private practice when your patient isn't progressing as well as you expected. Their recovery from injury might be slower than you initially told your patient, so to counteract this you give the patient more of your time.

Giving them a longer appointment slot serves to give you more time to try improving their symptoms within the session and at the same time you think you are doing them a favour by giving them what is in effect 'free' therapy. But they don't want more time; they just want you to improve their symptoms and get them back to full fitness.

If your sessions are continually running over, you also run the risk of upsetting your patients and your boss with appointment slots starting late or having to be cut short, because you can't manage your caseload and time well.

Some treatment slots can be as little as 30 minutes in private practice, so you need to have the ability to manage your time well. You need to be efficient with your assessment, hands-on treatments and rehab skills to get the necessary results with your patients so they get what they need (your intervention) within the allotted time slot.

Do you feel you are giving your patients value for money working in your private practice clinic?

Are they getting the best experience and is your level of care worthy of the £50/£60/£70 they are paying out of their hard-earned cash?

Once money is involved, the pressure and expectation increases tenfold to get patient results.

That is why many New Grads are put off by working in private practice and why some even more experienced therapists don't last long in this environment.

I've even known of qualified physiotherapists, sports therapists and sports rehabilitators who have downgraded their skill-sets and have chosen to operate as 'massage therapists' because they couldn't cope with the pressure and expectations that private practice brings.

They would rather just rub a client's lower back, hamstrings or whatever other area they have a problem with, because they don't have the belief in their own skill-sets to competently and confidently assess, treat and rehab patients, and feel overwhelmed trying to get them out of pain and back to full function.

It's such a shame to see therapists operating like this and is a complete waste of the time, effort and thousands of pounds spent working through their university-level education.

With all due respect, you can get a massage qualification over a weekend on any course that gives you the title and the authority to practice this way.

This is not how university-level therapists should be operating in private practice.

Getting Into Private Practice

Given the level of care expected and the pressure discussed above, employers in private practice often set a high bar on job applications.

Those that don't are often big therapy chains that operate on a mass scale, the same companies that have contracts with large government agencies or corporate firms or see most of their patients via private healthcare schemes.

These big companies operate on a mass level, often prioritising quantity over quality. I know many New Grad Physios who have felt overwhelmed by the sheer volume of patients seen per day.

They can be quite lucrative, particularly as a New Grad, but therapists often don't last that long in these environments as they feel their progression stagnates.

Whilst they are seeing many patients and getting the 'experience' and repetition of patients through the door, CPD and personal mentorship in these environments is often poor.

Therapists are often asked to work across multiple sites, almost always autonomously and lack the support they need when they get that tricky patient or they need help and support to keep learning and progressing their skills, both clinically and non-clinically.

Like therapists working in any domain, they then feel the need to pursue their own learning and CPD, often wasting hundreds, even thousands of pounds on evening and weekend courses to fill the void, only to be left feeling disappointed, frustrated and not able to apply their new-found learning.

In any full-time position, regardless of the setting, you should at least be getting weekly individual or group training, whether that is in the form of IST or scheduled paid teaching from your employer.

This is in addition to the access you should have to daily help and support from your senior colleagues and assigned mentor, as without this guidance your learning and progression will stagnate.

But most, if not all, offer no support; at best you might get a short monthly group IST session.

With any New Grad role, I can't stress enough how important it is to research who your senior therapists will be and what level of support is available to you daily.

You need to see past the pound signs and rather than money being the deciding factor to pursue a job or not, you should prioritise what learning opportunities that organisation can offer you.

You need to make sure the job pays well enough for you to live, pay your bills, rent, run your car etc, but your learning, and the support you get to progress your skills and your career must be paramount.

If you don't get the support you need, especially early in your career, you will not make the progress you need, and your journey to becoming a competent, confident and competitive New Grad Physio will be a long and challenging road.

In the short-term, it may hit you in the pocket, but you will make this back many times over in the future, as competent, confident and competitive therapists get paid more than their incompetent, unconfident and non-competitive peers.

Evening and Weekend Work

One of the downsides of private practice work is that you may be required to work evenings and weekends.

Whilst you will get the time off at other times in the working week, these hours are unsociable and can interfere with the rest of your life, hobbies, interests and social life.

You need to consider this when applying for such roles, and at the very least enquire how the working schedules are formulated and how much notice you receive if any changes are made.

What you want is to agree on set times and have a consistent working pattern, so you can then plan the other things you like to do outside of work.

Erratic working schedules make it difficult to plan your life outside of work which can leave you feeling overworked, frustrated and at the mercy of your job.

This is something that can be clarified once you have been offered the job, alongside negotiating contract terms and CPD allowances.

Autonomous Working

Working in private practice you will almost exclusively work autonomously.

Even working in a busy private clinic with multiple therapists, you can sometimes go hours without having a meaningful conversation with anyone other than your patients.

To offer maximum appointment availability to patients, lunch breaks are often staggered for staff, so even then you might not get to see and speak to your peers and co-workers.

This can be very different to an NHS or sporting environment whereby scheduled breaks are the same and the setup of working departments mean that you have increased engagement with your co-workers throughout the day.

Therefore, in private practice there is the risk that you can feel isolated and don't have anyone to turn to there and then when you need them.

My own rapid rise to the top, progressing from student to Head Physiotherapist in the Leeds Rhinos in a little over a year, left me feeling isolated and alone at times.

As a junior physio there was always someone to look up to, to support me and my learning, someone to bounce ideas off and ask questions when I needed, someone to double check a patient and give a second opinion, but now, as the lead physiotherapist I *was* that person.

Junior staff expected that of me, but I didn't have the same support myself. My mentor had left to pursue his own dream job, but I still needed support.

So, what I did was seek external mentorship and support; I paid to be mentored as I knew how important it was that I kept learning and progressing.

Yes, I had achieved my goal, my dream job, but I was humble enough and self-aware enough to know that there was so much more I didn't know and so much more I needed guidance with.

As you decide to pursue any therapy role the level of support offered is key if you want to progress your skill-sets and become a competent, confident and competitive New Grad Physio.

CHAPTER 11
How to excel working in professional sport as a New Grad Physio

Working in professional sport is very different to working within the NHS and private practice and like these environments brings its own challenges that are unique to this setting.

I was very clear in my own career path and always wanted to forge a career in professional sport, but I appreciate it's not for everyone. That said, many of the themes that are covered in this chapter can be applied to both private practice and the NHS so please read on.

As a New Grad, entering sport is often the hardest thing.

There are jobs available for New Grads but sometimes these are not always the best options. Whilst it will vary from sport to sport, many New Grad Physio roles involve work within sporting teams' academies and junior teams.

On the one hand these can be great environments to work in, often with much less pressure to win games and less pressure to push players quickly back from injury; on the other hand, these roles often require therapists to work autonomously and often off-site (schools, colleges etc).

Whilst a degree of autonomy is great for any New Grad, many of these environments don't have a good balance of autonomous practice and supervised practice.

Often New Grads find themselves working alone and don't have that support network of other therapists around them. They don't have someone working on the next plinth or in the next room to bounce ideas off or ask for a second clinical opinion. They lack guidance and support, and in many cases it shows.

Having worked with so many New Grads you can tell a big difference between those that have had good guidance and support in their early career and those that haven't.

Look at it like this…

If you are working in a department with other therapists, you can ask for advice there and then, watch and observe more experienced therapists at work and plan and work together at treatment and rehab sessions. If you're working autonomously you can't do any of these things.

So firstly, I would always consider the environment you are stepping into.

Does it have the level of support you need as a New Grad?

Are there other therapists you have access to when needed?

As good as a 'Head Of Academy' role might look on paper, always consider if it is the best job for you at that time.

One of the biggest compliments I have ever received was a therapist coming to work with me, mainly because he felt he'd be in a better environment to learn. He'd done some research and knew another therapist that I had worked with previously.

That therapist had suggested that at that time of his career he was better choosing opportunity and learning rather than pay.

He turned a job down that paid £5000 more, for in effect the same role, in the same sport, with the same hours and the same responsibilities. He chose it because he saw more value in his learning than short-term pay.

That therapist was in a junior role for only a couple of years before he successfully changed sports and got a role at his own dream job, working for Ireland's professional rugby union.

I myself can't speak more highly of the support and mentorship I received as a New Grad. Without question I would not have progressed so quickly up the promotion ladder had I not had that support. That aside, if you want to work in sport, or are already working in sport, there are some challenges unique to this environment.

So, what do you need to do to excel working in professional sport?

Understanding The Athlete Mindset

To be successful in professional sport we must first acknowledge that athletes can be very different 'patients' from those in private practice or the NHS.

The level of function they need to get back to and some of the external pressures they may be under (from themselves, teammates, fans, manager, media), their often-extensive previous injury history and possible contractual issues are just some of the unique characteristics that set athletes apart from the everyday patient.

But that's not what I want to highlight.

I want to emphasise how a global approach to athlete health and well-being is key to any management plan, and before we start designing any athlete management plan, we firstly must understand the athlete's mindset.

THE ATHLETE'S MIND

Working with any athlete brings its challenges least of all when a player is out injured. This is usually increased when an athlete is out for a considerable amount of time.

Many thoughts and emotions may run through an athlete's head when they are injured:

'Will I get back playing?'

'Will I have the same speed, footwork, strength and fitness that I had pre-injury?'

'Is this something that is going to continue to plague me during the rest of my career?

Each injury is different, and the severity and length of management will have a large impact on the possible emotions that an athlete might contend with.

Although it's not always the case, a player out for 4-6 weeks is less likely to have the same negative thought processes compared with a player out for 9-12 months. Either way, it is important that we as therapists first acknowledge that players can have these anxieties following injury, and second, we put interventions in place to ensure these issues don't impede the physical side of recovery from injury.

The more and more athletes I have seen the more and more I try delving into the psychological aspects of an injured athlete.

This side of rehab is something we are not taught in university, yet having worked in elite sport I know first-hand it must be addressed if you are going to have successful outcomes with your athletes.

There is now a growing awareness of mental or psychological health both within sport and in wider society. For therapists, this can only be a good thing, as our previous training hasn't prepared us to deal with the 'psychological' aspect of injury rehabilitation.

When working in elite rugby I had a long-term injured player suffering with depression. It was only flagged up once he had returned from injury and was back playing in the team.

I was truly surprised when he told me.

As a club we made sure he got the best possible care, but it didn't sit well with me. I had worked pretty much every day for the past nine months – he had sustained a major shoulder injury following an anterior shoulder dislocation. He had subsequent surgery, but recovery was slow as he had an associated neural injury as a result of the dislocation.

Keeping any player motivated and on track during a long-term injury is hard, and this player was no different. But his rehab process went well, we didn't have any setbacks and he returned to full shoulder function and successfully got back training and playing.

At no point did I think he was depressed. I thought I knew this player well; very well in fact. We had spent so much time together during this period, and had spoken about everything under the sun, yet I hadn't recognised that he needed help.

I was probably a bit naïve at this point of my career with regards to an athlete's mental health.

We can be like people looking from the outside in – we have the perception that athletes are strong, both physically and psychologically; they lead a good lifestyle, play a sport they probably grew up wanting to do and get a handsome pay packet for doing so.

All this can lead us to question what they have got to be depressed about.

This experience for me was a big eye-opener and led me to re-evaluate how I look at and plan the rehabilitation of an athlete. I am now conscious of both the physical and non-physical stressors, unique to sport, and can plan a package of care needed to give an athlete the support they need to make a successful return to sport.

To be able to do this and do this successfully we first need to…

Find Out Their 'WHAT'

First up we need to find out the **WHAT**. The big thing for me is finding out what players are worried about. This largely comes from being able to communicate well with your athletes and have a good understanding and rapport so that they are willing to divulge what anxieties and apprehensions they may have.

If you can get to the bottom of what is concerning your athlete, then you can put interventions in place. Without such information, you are just guessing.

We can write the best management and rehabilitation plan in the world but if any psychological issues are not addressed then we might not get the results we want and in the expected timeframe we want them. Previously such issues were largely a 'taboo' subject particularly within elite sports settings.

I have a background working extensively within rugby which is assumed to have rough, tough, robust athletes and personalities. But this is not always the case.

At the top level of their sport, rugby players face a great amount of pressure to perform. When they are injured and that right to play is taken away from them, some athletes struggle. They often feel they lack 'purpose', and why wouldn't they – whilst injured they can no longer do what they do and often feel they are letting themselves and other people down.

What has been beneficial recently is the great increase in the exposure mental health has been getting, both in sport and wider society. Current and past athletes speaking out about their own struggles with mental health will hopefully see mental health as no longer a taboo subject.

One athlete I worked with previously used his own personal battle with depression, which ran alongside him being injured and unable to play, to launch an online magazine, aiming to lift the lid on mental health and in turn help fellow athletes and the wider society. He speaks very openly about his own battles and has also interviewed several other athletes in relation to mental health issues.

This increased exposure can only be a good thing as it gets people engaged and talking about mental health and raises awareness of this important subject.

What is important is that you don't make assumptions that just because an athlete has a long-term injury, they will have a mental health issue that needs addressing and needs medical input.

This is firstly not true and, secondly, such assumptions will likely lead to generic interventions that are unlikely to find and manage the true stressor(s) for each individual athlete.

How individuals deal with injuries and 'stress' will differ greatly. Psychological well-being could be affected by their home life, relationships, contract negotiations or indeed any other aspect of their life, including injury.

If we do highlight issues, putting interventions in place is key – but these cannot be generic.

You need to find out what everyone wants and why they want it.

Matching Athlete Wants

As a therapist working with athletes, we want the athletes' needs and wants to align as closely as possible with our intervention goals. Giving the athletes some of what **THEY** want and getting from them what we need, will help ensure we reach the desired goal of the treatment plan.

If your intervention goals and your athlete's goals differ, you may need to spend some time educating your athlete of the purpose of your interventions.

If they can clearly see why you want to achieve those goals and how they relate to getting them to the end goal, athlete buy-in and adherence to your treatment plan will not be a problem.

In sport, we all want to build fit, skilful and robust athletes.

In a sporting setting, as practitioners we talk about robustness in terms of training or match availability whereas an athlete might talk in terms of match availability or even just being fit come the business end of the season and being ready for the 'big games'.

Whilst there are slight differences, both the sports practitioner and the athlete goals are along the same lines, but unless we connect the dots and establish the link between the two in the eyes of our athletes, then our interventions may fail.

I'm forever the optimist and like to view every injury as an **OPPORTUNITY**. The bigger the injury, the bigger that opportunity will be. That's the way you should try to sell it to the athletes you work with.

This is not a conversation you will be having on day one post-injury, but once the dust has settled and the athlete has got their head around their diagnosis and prognosis then it is advantageous to have that chat.

I like to speak to the athlete directly and ask them for individual goals in the following categories:

1 Physical Goals

2 Psychological Goals

3 Non-Athletic Goals

With any injury, there are always other physical goals we can tailor into our management plan. We can address issues we might have picked up on their movement screening or prioritise other developments the athlete and/or the strength and conditioning team want to pursue. This helps us to focus and gives the athlete some control to their training and rehab aims which will aid athlete buy-in.

Athletes might sometimes be reluctant to list psychological goals, but this is far and away becoming a thing of the past. Some athletes just need a nudge and to be asked the right questions. If they have a good level of trust and rapport with us then they will express any issues they have.

Setting non-athletic goals often helps the overall management plan. It gives athletes an external focus and can ensure they feel they are making progress, even if that might be in another part of their lives.

Within the last year some of the athletes I have worked with have engaged with university study, music lessons, blogging and much more. All these athletes might not have proceeded in this way if we hadn't sat down and discussed such goal setting. **ALL** these athletes have also reported that these non-athletic goals were highly advantageous in helping them come back stronger, both physically and mentally, following long-term injury.

To give the tools needed to overcome the challenges they face, we firstly need to identify each individual athlete's issues, making sure to account for both physical and psychological factors. Secondly, we need to put interventions in place that reflect that individual's issues to maximise buy-in, ensuring our interventions align closely with the needs and wants of our athletes.

In doing so we can ensure athletes reduce the risk of developing non-physical issues which can positively influence their physical recovery from injury.

Further Pressures Of A 'Results-Driven' Industry

Professional sport is a results-driven industry. For that reason, there is massive pressure on medical staff to supply the coaches with their best players to give them the best opportunity to practice and in turn be available for as many games as possible.

These pressures commonly see therapists making mistakes and pushing players too hard; this is one of the main reasons we see high re-injury rates within professional sport.

Each injury has individual circumstances and as a result individual decision-making for each patient is different.

How you might manage a player with a low-grade hamstring injury might be different in different situations. If it was the last game of the season and it was a Cup Final, or a game to stop that team being relegated, then this is very different to a preseason friendly or weekly normal competition fixture.

There is always a risk-reward decision to be made with any athlete with regards to their availability to both train and play, and each decision should be made on a case-by-case basis.

What is very important, however, is that you have the confidence that the athlete is ready in the first place to return.

The pressure of sport often causes therapists to skip steps in order to rush players back. I'm sure you have seen things like 'Accelerated ACL Programmes' or similar programmes for many other sporting injuries. No programme can be accelerated, and no programme should be time based.

As a therapist you need a step-by-step system that you take every athlete or patient through, which is logical and systematic and gets your athlete back on the field of play without the fear of injury returning, regardless of the injury they present with.

We spoke during the last chapter about private practice patients who drop off after sessions 2 or 3, having much improved symptoms, but many get back to their desired activities too quickly and many break down again. Athletes are no different, although, in this case, we (the therapist) are consciously succumbing to the pressure and skipping steps, not taking athletes through a full graded rehab plan and in turn are contributing to the high level of re-injury rates we see within professional sport.

Any athlete or patient needs that graded exposure to exercise. Skipping steps to try and shave a few days off an injury doesn't give them that graded exposure and the time their body often needs to adapt between each progression. That is why system-led care, and logical and systematic step-by-step treatment plans win every time over 'accelerated' style treatment plans.

It looks fantastic if you get a six-week injury back in three weeks, but if they break down in the first minute of their first game back it doesn't look so good!

Not only will your athletes lose faith in you, so will the head coach or manager, who will question your decision-making and ability to deal with working with athletes in such a high-pressure environment.

The best therapists I have ever worked with nail the basics.

They don't follow trends or treatment fads and don't always have extensive training in specialist areas; they just do the basics extraordinarily well.

Most therapists will go full circle in their careers, in the sense that they will go on weekend 'specialist' training courses, spend £1000s on CPD, spending many years working and experimenting trying to find the best way to assess, treat and rehab their athletes and patients, only to realise they get the best results by doing basic things really well.

That's almost the best thing about being a New Grad Physio. You are a blank canvas and have the opportunity right **NOW** to create a path for your own learning and development. You can choose to learn a proven treatment system right **NOW** and get the guidance you need to become a competent, confident and competitive New Grad Physio or choose to spend the next five to ten years struggling, trying to work this out on your own.

CHAPTER 12
A day in the life of a New Grad Physio

As we come towards the later chapters in this book, it is important we take stock and acknowledge the journey any New Grad Physio must make transitioning out of university and into the real world.

Even if you are a student and not quite facing these challenges, the content in this book alone will have highlighted the big challenges that you will face in your quest to become a competent, confident and competitive New Grad Physio.

If you have already graduated you will no doubt be fighting these challenges head-on, right now.

Regardless of your current situation, despite the challenges you face, I don't want you to feel overwhelmed.

The main purpose of this book is to help New Grad Physios just like you to identify the challenges that you will face and give you some solutions to the most common problems.

Failing to overcome these challenges makes your life as a New Grad therapist difficult and unenjoyable.

However, meeting these problems head-on and overcoming them gives you the chance to become that competent and confident New Grad Physio, to enjoy your role, get the patient results you want and become competitive enough to start climbing the promotion ladder.

I know from my own personal experiences as a New Grad how hard this stage of your professional career can be. Having worked and coached so many other New Grads through the same challenges at this stage of their own professional careers has only confirmed this.

But life as a therapist can be so rewarding and satisfying, knowing that you have the skills to be able to help people, your patients, out of pain and back to full function and to make a meaningful impact on their lives.

That's massive!

Getting a patient back in the gym or running, helping another get back to work ASAP so that they can provide for their family, helping another out of pain so he or she can get back gardening or playing with their grandkids, fills you with pride and accomplishment.

Not many jobs are this rewarding; we just need to be sure we can come up with the goods and get the positive patient results that we and our patients desire.

Becoming the next competent, confident and competitive New Grad Physio requires hard work and effort and the right support network.

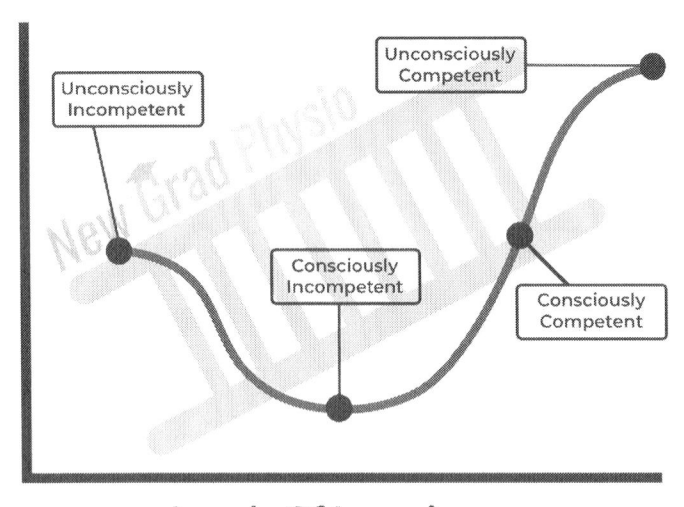

Levels Of Learning

Figure 5 – New Grad Physio Competency Ladder. Adapted from (Burch, 1970)

How To Get Noticed and Gain Entry To Your First Role In The NHS, Private Practice or Sport – Competency 1

At the first stage of the New Grad Physio Competency Ladder therapists are operating as 'Unconsciously Incompetent'; this relates particularly to student therapists.

The biggest challenge therapists face at this stage is the lack of awareness about the challenges that are on the horizon as 'You Don't Know What You Don't Know'. As hard as you think the challenges of combining studies with placements are, the real challenges you will face as a New Grad Physio are yet to start.

Promising therapists are blissfully unaware of these challenges and equally lack the awareness that the decisions they make at this stage have such a major bearing on what will happen later in their professional careers.

It's the challenge of the unknown and the challenge to identify the barriers and the problems that they will face in the future and to act early.

Gaining entry to the workplace into the area you would like to work is challenging. There are jobs out there, but if you have ambition, drive and goals, you shouldn't have to accept any job, just to get started.

When you've spent years at university and worked hard to get to this point, do you really want to accept a mediocre role? I didn't and you shouldn't either. The key to being successful at this stage is learning how to get noticed and gain entry.

Regardless of whether you want to pursue a career in the NHS, private practice or sport, at this stage you need to learn three key things:

  1 How to set clear career goals.

  2 How to identify what barriers are stopping you achieving your goals and what you can do to break these barriers.

  3 How to stand out from the crowd and avoid selling yourself short.

Failure to do these three key things may stop your career in its tracks before it has even started.

Unfortunately, just sending a CV in and landing your dream New Grad role doesn't happen. You must be strategic about how you do this.

You need clear career goals that give your actions intent, remembering that a lack of intent causes a lack of results.

You need to acknowledge that some barriers you cannot affect and as such you shouldn't lose time and effort on these. Instead you should focus on controlling the controllable factors to maximise your path towards your desired career goal.

You need to make sure your 'dream job' is really your 'dream job' and you can do this by test driving this role to see if it is really for you; otherwise, you are just guessing.

The best candidates do not always get the best roles. Those that can showcase their skills and those that don't sell themselves short in the eyes of their potential employers are those that get the best roles. We covered all these challenges and some solutions to these back in Chapter 5.

Navigating the job market, entering the workforce in a role you truly want and progressing up the promotion ladder is no easy feat.

Whether you are looking at securing your first job following graduation or trying to get ahead as a student, being successful in gaining entry is all about making opportunities for yourself and being ready to grasp these opportunities with both hands once they present themselves.

How To SURVIVE As A New Grad Physio – Competency 2

I have yet to meet a New Grad Physio who felt fully prepared post-university to deal with the challenges of working with real patients in the real world, myself included.

At this point the majority of New Grads fully appreciate the enormity of the challenges they face and how big the knowledge gap really is between what they learned at university and what is required to be a successful New Grad in the real world.

The knowledge and skills gap is scary and it's no wonder it makes you feel incompetent, overwhelmed, frustrated and even angry; I remember those feelings like it was yesterday.

This 'Ah-ha' moment relates to Competency 2 on the New Grad Physio Competency Ladder as New Grads become 'Consciously Incompetent'.

Despite now being a fully-fledged and 'qualified' therapist, you feel less equipped and ready to deal with your patients than you did when you were still a student. And unless you do something about it you will continue to struggle or at best will just be able to keep your head above water in a busy and challenging medical department.

This is highlighted by the drop in the level of learning shown on the New Grad Physio Competency Ladder.

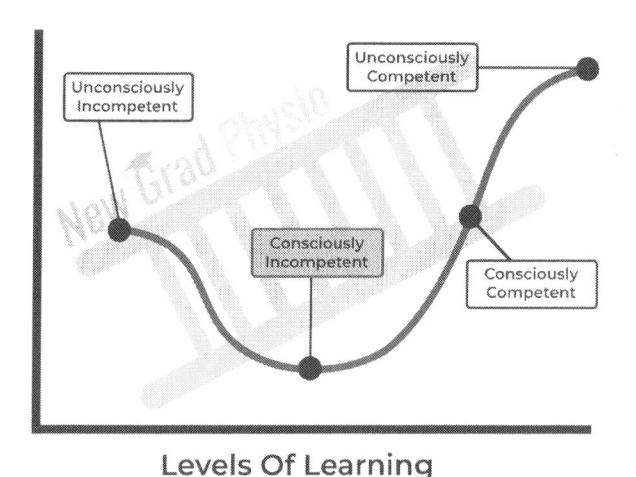

Levels Of Learning

Figure 6 – Stage 2 'Consciously Incompetent' New Grad Physio Competency Ladder. Adapted from (Burch, 1970)

Whilst you are now qualified and no longer a student, the increased pressure and expectations at this stage, and the knowledge gap between what you were taught at university and what you need to know to get positive patient results means that you actually regress.

You are exposed to an environment that you haven't been prepared for.

You are seeing some injuries and pathologies for the first time.

You have shorter appointment slots and no longer have the support of your clinical educator or university lecturer by your side.

You are now qualified, which means your patients and your senior colleagues expect you to get your patients better.

Yet, your studies didn't prepare you for these challenges.

At this stage you must learn and learn quickly if you are to SURVIVE as a New Grad Physio. Central to being able to SURVIVE at this stage is learning:

- How to manage a busy clinical caseload.
- How to understand your patient assessments and extract the 'useful' from the 'useless' information from both your subjective and objective assessments.
- How to design a full treatment and rehab plan and take a patient through it – from start to finish.

The challenge of shorter treatment slots and higher patient and senior staff expectations means that you need to be time efficient whilst still getting results.

You need to be able to manage your own caseloads, ensuring that appointments run on time. Running over can leave you feeling rushed and flustered, and you can miss important patient information during your assessments.

You need to understand the 'what' and 'why' of your patient assessments to help you choose the correct hands-on treatment techniques and rehab exercises to get your patients out of pain and back to full function.

Your university teachings taught you a basic patient assessment, meaning you may miss important patient information that might be the difference between you being able to make quick changes to your patient symptoms and struggling to make any changes at all.

You need to screen for important information, like red flags, but, more important than that, you need to know what to do if a patient answers YES to these questions.

Do you know what the next step is if a patient FAILS your red flag questions? Don't worry if you don't, most other New Grad Physios don't know either.

You also need to know how to take a patient from the clinic bed and back to full function by designing and implementing an effective treatment plan.

University left us with very few hands-on treatment techniques and rehab exercises to choose from.

I quickly learnt that those Maitland mobilisations, NAGs and SNAGs and McKenzie style exercises didn't work for most patients I was working with. They didn't get these patients out of pain like my university lecturers told me they would.

I was left feeling incompetent and inadequate and struggling to survive as a New Grad Physio. I've no doubt you feel the same, as you worry about the next patient who walks through your door and question yourself whether you have the hands-on skills to deal with their problems.

Your busy days in hospital, the clinic or the long days working in sport leave you feeling frustrated at the lack of time you are spending on your continued learning and CPD.

You feel like you are falling behind some of your peers and your knowledge and learning is stagnating.

You are not able to keep up-to-date with the latest research and can no longer find the time to read journal articles like you did whilst at university.

Time is our most precious resource and unlike other resources we unfortunately cannot make more of it.

You can't make more hours in the day but what you can do is find other ways to digest content that will give you the skill-sets needed to SURVIVE as a New Grad Physio. This content needs to be of a high quality, accessible and concise given the constraints on your time working in a busy medical department.

How To Not Only Survive But THRIVE As A New Grad Physio – Competency 3

The next progression for any New Grad Physio is becoming 'Consciously Competent' which represents Stage 3 on the New Grad Physio Competency Ladder.

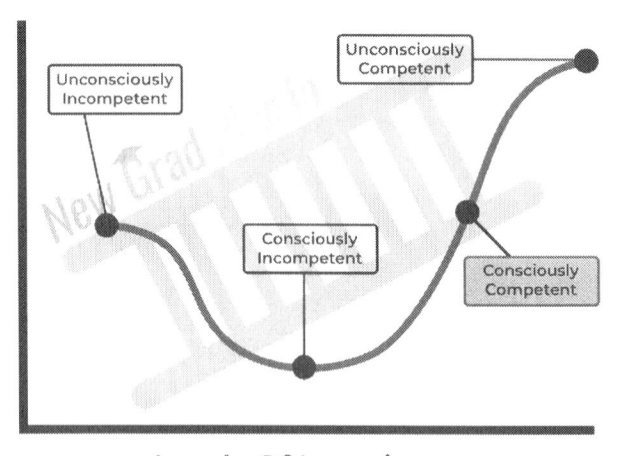

Levels Of Learning

Figure 7 – Stage 3 'Consciously Competent' New Grad Physio Competency Ladder. Adapted from (Burch, 1970)

This stage relates to a therapist working as a Band 5 in the NHS, just starting out in private practice or working at 'Academy' level in sport.

At Stage 3, New Grad Physios are starting to build some proficiency in their practice, with some basic skills becoming more automatic.

But as you progress, you will be given more responsibility, feel more pressure and experience greater levels of expectation from both your patients and your senior colleagues.

The skills-sets required at this stage, those we covered in Chapter 7, require improved clinical skills and non-clinical skills, as you continue your path towards becoming that competent, confident and competitive New Grad Physio.

Key to success at Stage 3 and becoming 'Consciously Competent' is learning:

- How to gain the trust, respect and recognition you deserve from both your patients and senior colleagues.
- How to build rapport with your patients and how to communicate effectively with both your patients and senior colleagues.
- How to get patients to adhere to your treatment plans and actually get better.

The reality of the challenges at this stage leave New Grad Physios still feeling like their patients look at them as young and inexperienced therapists.

Whilst you may be able to build some proficiency in your clinical skills at this stage, your lack of ability to gain trust, build rapport and communicate your clinical message clearly is affecting patient buy-in and adherence to your treatment plans.

You feel you lack the confidence and authority a qualified therapist should have, and this is affecting your ability to make positive changes to patient symptoms.

This is a real 'Ouch' moment for many New Grad therapists.

Having navigated the first weeks and months as a New Grad Physio (Stage 2) you thought things would get easier, but for many the challenges get bigger and more difficult.

Despite your qualified status you feel you lack 'REAL' responsibility; you are not taken seriously and are not confident to give input in MDT meetings or to put your neck on the line by making important clinical decisions.

You feel you are not getting the support you need to progress your career and upskill in areas you know you need to develop.

You lack direction as to what you should be focusing your learning on and direction as to what CPD options might be beneficial to your own practice and development.

You've maybe even wasted your time and money on evening and weekend courses that appeared helpful at the time, but have left you feeling disappointed, as you have been unable to apply this knowledge to your practice and have cost you significant investment financially.

Even at this stage, therapists can feel overwhelmed with regards to their patient assessments, hands-on treatment techniques and rehab planning.

Added to this is the challenge of building trust, gaining the respect and recognition you deserve, and communicating your clinical message effectively to patients so they no longer see you as that young and inexperienced therapist, but start buying into and adhering to your treatment plans.

If you lack these skills, patients will not trust what you are telling them to do, they will not adhere to your treatment plans, and you will continue to be an incompetent therapist, in the eyes of both your patients and senior colleagues.

Getting Your Next Promotion – Competency 4

The final step of the New Grad Physio Competency Ladder is Stage 4 when therapists become 'Unconsciously Competent'. Having gained clarity and proficiency in their clinical skills, they start to gain the belief they can progress and move up the promotion ladder.

At this stage on a clinical level being 'Unconsciously Competent' means therapists are starting to build towards 'mastery', whereby their clinical skills start to become second nature.

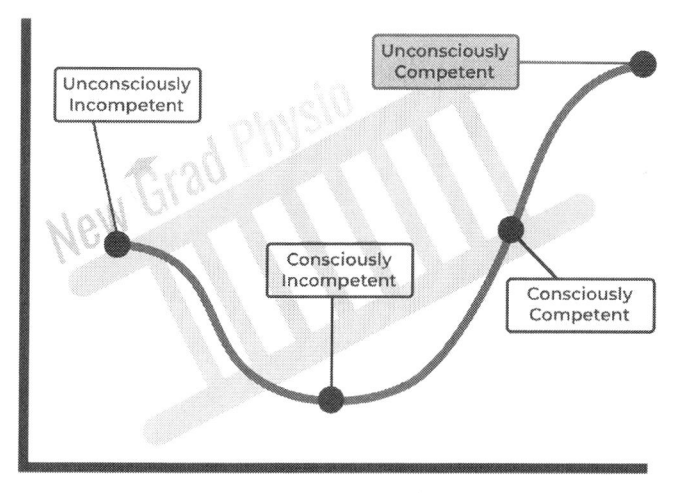

Levels Of Learning

Figure 8 – Stage 4 'Unconsciously Competent' New Grad Physio Competency Ladder. Adapted from (Burch, 1970)

At this stage you might start to 'specialise' in an area, consistently seeing more complex caseloads, planning and implementing higher level treatment and rehab plans and gaining more responsibilities within your working department.

This stage would reflect a therapist working at Band 6 level in the NHS, an autonomous private practice therapist or a therapist working at first team level within a sports setting.

The complexity of patient caseloads increases at this stage, added to further responsibilities including supporting and mentoring others i.e. junior staff, leading training (IST sessions) and having more input with organisational and managerial tasks.

At this stage you need more clarity in your assessments as you deal with more complex patients and are now regarded as a 'specialist' in this area. You need the skill-sets to start being able to find the true source of patient symptoms, rather than just managing them, in order to stop patients regressing and their symptoms returning.

You need the skills to be able to manage other people and to mentor and support others, whilst still ensuring you continue to progress your own knowledge base and the application of this knowledge.

Despite moving up the promotion ladder, many therapists at this stage still question their abilities as a therapist, their ability to operate as a 'specialist' and often feel that they are in a 'false' position and are not actually as good as they thought.

Whilst a progression in responsibility is what you wanted you may still feel inadequate to deal with some of the new challenges that present themselves.

You lack the real belief in your ability to 'specialise' and are left frustrated when you can't get more complex patients out of pain.

You've heard that the site and source of symptoms are different, and you know that you need to be able to identify a patient's 'true stressor' if you are to take away their pain and stop that pain from returning.

You are dealing with patients who have failed under the care of other therapists and have been referred to you as a 'specialist', yet you lack the skills to get a positive patient outcome.

It is common at this point for therapists to transition from one area to another, moving in or out of roles in the NHS, private practice or sport, wrongly assuming these environments are different.

But whilst the environments are different the same challenges are still there.

To become a competent, confident and competitive New Grad Physio and truly become a therapist operating at Stage 4 as 'Unconscious Competent' you need to nail how to deal with complex patient caseloads, programme and implement higher level rehab and have the skills to manage and mentor junior staff.

To even get to this stage and be promoted to higher level roles in the first place is a big challenge. The lack of skills to put together a great CV and nail your interview means that moving up the promotion ladder is much more difficult than you thought.

Key to success at Stage 4, becoming 'Unconsciously Competent' and gaining that next promotion, is learning:

- How to write a knockout therapy CV
- How to smash your interview making it virtually impossible for employers to turn you down
- How to make opportunities happen and how to fly up the promotion ladder faster than you ever thought possible

Whilst therapists at this stage are skilled, those that can climb the promotion ladder are those who acknowledge they need additional support and specialist skills to progress.

Whether that is moving up within an existing or similar organisation or transitioning from one area of therapy to another, you need to nail the above skills and learn how to create further opportunities for yourself to move up the promotion ladder and a step closer to your dream role.

I'm sure you can relate to each step on the New Grad Physio Competency Ladder and place yourself somewhere along that journey.

Even if you perceive yourself to be at one of the later stages on the ladder, you will have missed some important steps that are likely holding you back from becoming that competent, confident and competitive New Grad Physio.

Can you honestly say that you are happy in your current position?

Do you know where your career is heading and have a plan in place to climb the promotion ladder towards your dream job?

Do you have the complete clarity in your patient assessments, hands-on treatment techniques and rehab planning to deal with any patient who walks through your clinic door?

Are you able to build rapport and trust with your patients and communicate your clinical findings effectively so that patients adhere to your treatment plans and complete every rep of every set of their home exercise programme?

Are you ready to take on more responsibility and want to further progress your career but are stuck and don't understand why you are not being selected for interview or, if you are getting interviews, why you are not being offered the job?

Do you feel you lack the skills to write a proper therapy CV, unsure how to make it professional, nail your 'pitch', and present your skills and attributes on paper? Or are you unsure how to showcase these same attributes in person during interview? Do you feel the lack of these skills is stopping you climbing the promotion ladder at the speed you should be?

If you are ready to become the next competent, confident and competitive New Grad Physio, have the ambition to be the best therapist you can be, providing the highest level of care to your patients and want to progress up the promotion ladder faster than you ever thought possible, keep reading…

CHAPTER 13
The fastest way to becoming a competent, confident and competitive New Grad Physio

Right now, you have a decision to make…

You can choose to follow the 'traditional' pathway, spend the next five to ten years as a frustrated and overwhelmed therapist trying to make sense of your patient assessments, trying to improve your hands-on treatment techniques and rehab planning, with the feeling you are not progressing your learning and your career at the rate you want.

Or, you can choose to act, save yourself years of feeling frustrated and overwhelmed by learning exactly how to become a competent, confident and competitive New Grad Physio. Unless you act, your goal, aspiration or dream job will not get any closer as you lack the support you need to make it a reality and not just a pipe-dream.

Whilst the NHS, private practice and sport have their unique challenges, the biggest mistake New Grad Physios make, regardless of the area they work, is not making the maximum use of their first few years upon graduating.

This is the primary time to make the biggest improvements in your skills, both clinically and non-clinically, and it's easy. With the right support you can become that competent, confident and competitive New Grad Physio and climb up the promotion ladder faster than you ever thought possible.

I designed the New Grad Physio Membership for exactly this reason. The content is specific to address the actual challenges you are facing as a New Grad Physio and gives you the help and guidance you need, the solutions you need, to overcome these challenges.

This is a programme built for New Grad Physios and New Grad Physios only.

I have created a learning platform for therapists like you, therapists who have the desire and potential to succeed, but need help and guidance to start getting those consistent, positive patient results. It will teach you how to get your patients to adhere to their treatment plans, to gain the trust and respect of your senior colleagues to get that next promotion and to maximise your potential.

I remember as a New Grad Physio there was always something that would be running through my mind and sometimes be keeping me awake at night. It was a difficult patient or athlete I was struggling with and who was booked in the next day. It was the anxiety about what I would do if he or she presented with similar symptoms, or worse, if their symptoms had regressed. It was the uncertainty about what I should be reading and what I should be spending my time learning to make myself a better therapist without wasting my time, effort and money.

I was lucky that I had the support and mentorship of a physio who had been through all these challenges himself and could guide me to avoid making the same mistakes, and the bigger consequences that he had made.

I was able to fast-track my learning and skillsets enabling me to achieve my dream job little over a year out of university, a job I was told would take my 10+ years to achieve.

I was driven, I had worked hard to get to that point, but I would never have been able to progress so quickly without the help and guidance I got as a New Grad Physio.

I now want to give you the same help and guidance I received to guide you on your own New Grad journey.

Are you ready to act and join the community of New Grad therapists already fast-tracking their own careers and learning the skill-sets needed to become the next competent, confident and competitive New Grad Physio?

What You Will Get When You Join The New Grad Physio Membership

Once inside the New Grad Physio Membership you will get exclusive access to content that specifically helps you overcome every challenge you will face as you progress through your New Grad Physio journey.

The content will include clinical modules on patient assessments, both subjective and objective, and hands-on treatment techniques and rehabilitation strategies that are proven to work in the real world, helping you attain real results with your patients.

Specific modules will also cover goal setting and career guidance, building rapport and trust with your patients and senior colleagues, how to communicate effectively, how to get patients to adhere to your treatment plan and how to get your next promotion.

The blend of clinical and non-clinical content will give you ALL the skill-sets you need to gain competency, build confidence, be successful and at the same time start enjoying your life as a New Grad Physio.

The overall programme is built to last 49 weeks, 1 week to consume the Introductory Bonus Content followed by 12 monthly teaching blocks.

Each monthly teaching block will focus on two body areas and over the course of the programme will cover the ankle, knee, hip, lumbar spine, cervical spine and shoulder. Each teaching block will upskill you on key subjective and objective assessment techniques, hands-on treatment techniques and rehab exercises specific to that body area.

At the end of each monthly block you will receive a quiz, helping you to consolidate the content you have covered and to ensure clarity and understanding of the material. Completion of the quiz will unlock a specific Bonus Module. These Bonus Modules directly link to skill-sets you need specific to each stage of your development and relate directly to the stages of the New Grad Physio Competency Ladder.

Additional to the content within the New Grad Physio Community portal you will have full access to the Private New Grad Physio Members Only Facebook Group. This group provides a platform for you to ask questions and get help 24/7 from both myself and other New Grad Physios in the same position as you. These could be questions relating to a problem patient or tricky injury you might be struggling with.

I post weekly real-life case studies in this private group, giving you exposure to injuries and their management that you might not see otherwise. Early in the week I present each case study in the group, before presenting my clinical thought process at the end of the week. The intervening period allows you to test yourself and to determine your diagnosis and prognosis and how you would manage the same injury. This allows you to think and work through a clinical reasoning process without having the pressure of a real-life patient in your clinic room.

I also post recent and must-read journal articles in the group as part of the 'New Grad Physio Book Club', saving you the time looking for this content yourself and expensive journal subscription costs.

You also have input into the topic of each month's 'Monthly Masterclass', a 20- to 30-minute webinar I stream live into the Facebook group each month. I post a poll of possible topics into the private group, all members vote, and the topic with the most votes wins. As the webinar runs live you can ask any questions during the webinar. But don't worry if you can't catch the webinar live; I record them all, so you can catch up at a time convenient to you.

At the end of each month I will send you a cheat sheet that will summarise the content of the monthly teaching block, helping you consolidate the content and giving you a quick reference guide to refer to.

In less than one year (49 weeks to be exact), with a small amount of weekly time commitment (less than 15 minutes per week) I can take you from your current position as a struggling, overwhelmed, incompetent and unskilled therapist into a competent, confident and competitive New Grad Physio, who is able to get consistently great patient results.

You can upskill this quickly, if you choose to act and invest in the right guidance and support as opposed to following the same path most other therapists take and reach the same level in five to ten years' time.

As you progress through the New Grad Physio Competency Ladder, the content changes to ensure you have the necessary skill-sets to overcome the challenges that are facing you right at that time.

You probably have a lot of questions about the New Grad Physio Membership and want to find out more. For that reason, I have put together some information below that you will find helpful.

Who Is The New Grad Physio?

The New Grad Physio is Andy Barker, consultant physiotherapist and private practice owner. Andy is currently providing consultancy to the Football Association both domestically and internationally. Andy also consults within a variety of other professional sports alongside lecturing on a variety of BSc and MSc therapy courses around the country.

What Does The New Grad Physio Aim To Do?

The New Grad Physio Membership aims to quicken the transition between university and the real world and give you the knowledge and skill-sets needed to become a competent, confident and competitive New Grad Physio. The programme is solely designed for New Grad Physios just like you, teaching you the missing modules university didn't teach you and teaching you what you **Need To Know** to be successful. The New Grad Physio does NOT show you what the textbooks and journals tell you works but shows you what works in the real world.

The New Grad Physio Membership teaches New Grad Physios the **three Cs,** enabling them to become **Competent, Confident and Competitive** New Grad Physios.

A New Grad Physio who is **Competent** has the clinical skill-sets needed to understand their patient assessments, provide hands-on treatment and prescribe rehab exercises that take away a patient's pain and get them back to full function.

A New Grad Physio who is **Confident** can easily build patient rapport, gain respect and recognition from their patients and senior staff and can communicate their clinical messages well so patients believe what they are saying and adhere to their treatment plans.

A New Grad Physio who is **Competitive** can stand out from the crowd, get ahead of their peers to get the jobs they want and fly up the promotion ladder faster than anyone thought possible.

Is The New Grad Physio For Me?

We have New Grad Physiotherapists, Sports Therapists and Sports Rehabilitators inside the New Grad Physio Membership.

The New Grad Physio Membership is taught in such a way that skills are transferable and can be applied to any setting, regardless of whether you work in the NHS, private practice or sport.

The programme will include some content that will be more appropriate to higher level and athletic populations who need exposure to higher loads but the progressions to this point are the same.

Do I Need To Be Qualified To Be Part Of The New Grad Physio Membership?

No, you don't. We understand that many therapists want to get ahead of the game and therefore we welcome both qualified and student therapists. The content is delivered in a way that will simplify many complex themes and as such is appropriate for both student and qualified therapists.

The Content Sounds Complicated, Is It Difficult To Apply?

Whilst the challenges as a New Grad Physio are difficult, the content is not. The New Grad Physio system teaches you a logical common-sense approach, giving you the structure you need to apply the evidence base and get the positive patient results you want.

The content is easy to follow and the monthly 'Cheat Sheets' I provide summarise the main teaching points and provide a quick reference guide to refer back to whenever you need them, taking the stress out of your day-to-day practice.

How Much Time Do I Need To Commit Each Week?

I appreciate that every person learns at his/her own pace. I also appreciate that life can also get in the way of you trying to spend time on your own learning. I know that trying to commit several hours a week to CPD is unrealistic and is a major barrier most New Grad Physios attribute to their learning stagnating. I know how frustrating it is spending hours and hours watching learning content only to pick up one or two things that you can apply.

For that very reason, I have designed the membership to deliver weekly content that will take you less than 15 minutes to consume. If you can commit to just 15 minutes per week, the New Grad Physio Membership will provide you with concise, quality content that you can apply straight away with your patients and athletes.

Just to keep you on track, I send out a weekly email reminder that lets you know the new weekly content has just been uploaded to the learning portal.

Additional to the weekly content, you will unlock bonus modules as you complete each month's content. These bonus modules are constantly being updated and as such each individual module will vary in length.

What Happens When I Sign Up?

Upon signing up you will receive an email immediately with your login details welcoming you to the New Grad Physio Membership. In this email you will also receive a link to join the Private 'Members Only New Grad Physio Facebook Group' (more about this later). Once inside the New

Grad Physio Membership learning portal you can get working through the content straight away.

Is All Content Delivered Via Webinars?

Unlike many online courses, content in the New Grad Physio Membership is delivered via various media methods. The New Grad Physio team have found that members find the best online learning experience contains a mixture of webinar presentations, practical tutorial videos, Facebook Lives, exercise demonstrations and individual online coaching calls. The Members Only New Grad Physio Facebook Group also adds another level of interaction where you can ask questions 24/7 to clarify the programme content or ask any specific questions about your own learning. At the completion of each month's content you will receive a 'Cheat Sheet' which will summarise the main content points of the previous month's teaching.

What Are Coaching Calls?

Coaching calls are one-to-one video calls with one of the New Grad Physio team where you can ask specific questions about the specific challenges you are struggling with. They are designed to provide individual support to you and to complement the New Grad Physio Membership content and the support given within the Members Only New Grad Physio Facebook Group.

What Happens When Membership Content Is Updated In The Future?

Medicine continues to evolve, and the evidence base you use to guide your practice is constantly changing. Andy is constantly updating content to match the changing needs of you as a New Grad Physio, striving to deliver easier ways for you to apply your skills and become that competent, confident and competitive New Grad Physio. As a member you will have instant and full access to any updates made to the content, including any additional bonuses added to the membership.

Do I Have To Attend In Person To Be Part Of This Members Group?

Not at all. All content is delivered online via a mixture of webinar presentations, practical tutorial videos, Facebook lives, exercise demonstrations and online coaching calls. All video footage is filmed in a videography studio, providing you with top quality content, ensuring we deliver an exceptional learning experience to you as a New Grad Physio member and allowing you to access the content at times that work around your own working and social schedule.

Do I Have To Sign Up For a Certain Period Or Can I Cancel At Any Time?

You are not tied into a lengthy membership and you can cancel at any time. There is a quick form in your members account page and that will let us know you want to cancel your subscription. This will take effect immediately and no further payment will be taken.

Why Does Enrolment Only Open At Certain Points In The Year?

So we can provide the best learning experience for members within the New Grad Physio Membership, Andy only opens enrolment at certain times a year. This is so Andy and the New Grad Physio team can give you our full attention and the high level of support you need to consume the New Grad Physio Membership content. In addition, if members start and work through the content at specific time points, it helps us to answer common questions and provide any additional content that might be needed during key stages of the programme.

Will I Be Able To Use This Learning Towards My CPD?

Yes. At the completion of each stage of competency of the New Grad Physio Competency Ladder you will receive a CPD certificate showing your proof of attendance. You can use these certificates to put towards your CPD training.

Why Is This Programme Different To Others?

The New Grad Physio Membership is different to a weekend course or other online training as it's not just about improving your subjective, objective, hands-on treatment skills and rehab planning. It is about understanding WHY you are asking certain subjective questions and understanding WHAT you are trying to achieve with your hands-on treatment and rehab planning. It gives you the skill-sets needed to learn how to build patient rapport and buy-in to your treatment plans and gain the trust and respect you deserve from your patients, peers and senior colleagues. The content helps you set career goals and gives you the direction and the skills needed to get your next promotion and work towards your own dream job.

It gives you an accessible and continued support network that doesn't finish once the course ends, like an evening or weekend course does. This allows the opportunity to ask questions and to access additional material that is relevant to the challenges you are facing right at that time.

The New Grad Physio Membership is a purpose-built learning platform specifically for New Grad Physios with the sole goal of helping you gain the competence and confidence in your practice you need to become a competitive and successful New Grad Physio.

If you have any further questions not covered above, please reach out to me using the contact details at the start and end of this book.

Still On The Fence?

The New Grad Physio Membership is perfect for you if you answer **YES** to any one of these questions:

- You are a student or qualified therapist and you are frustrated trying to get your first job.
- You feel like you lack a clear career plan and the support needed to

identify and overcome the barriers stopping you making progression towards your dream job.

- You are struggling to write a knockout CV to get you an interview or are unsure why you are not being offered a job having made the interview shortlist.

- You want to be able to provide a service to your patients you feel they deserve and to start enjoying your day-to-day practice as a New Grad.

- You have successfully got a job but feel like you are not getting the learning support you currently need to improve your skill-sets.

- You sometimes struggle to make sense of your patient assessments and feel like you need a better system to add structure to your assessments allowing you to extract the information you need to make positive patient outcomes.

- You feel university left you feeling unprepared to deal with the challenges as a New Grad Physio, and missed important information you now need to become a competent, confident and competitive therapist.

- You lack the ability to design and implement a full rehabilitation plan, and are unable to take a patient through a full course of treatment from the clinic bed back to full function.

- You struggle to build rapport with your patients, and you feel they just see you as a young and inexperienced therapist.

- You struggle to build trust with your patients, and some patients don't buy-in to your treatment plans, resulting in poor adherence, patient drop-offs and poor patient outcomes.

- You struggle to deliver your clinical message to your patients, and you feel they don't trust what you are saying.

- You lack the skills and confidence to deliver clinical information to your peers and senior colleagues and feel you are not given the respect you deserve as a qualified therapist.

- You want to make the next step in your career and move up the promotion ladder, but are not sure how to do this.
- You want proven methods that work in the real world and not just treatment techniques and rehab exercise the textbooks tell you work, but in reality don't.
- You are driven, motivated and enthusiastic about your learning and becoming the best New Grad Physio you can be.
- You don't want to waste your time, effort and money over the next five to ten years trying to 'figure this stuff out' or 'making numerous mistakes' on your own; instead you want real life results right NOW.
- You realise that you need guidance and support if you are to reach your full potential as a therapist (something I was extremely lucky to get at such an early point in my career).

If you answered YES to any of the above questions and if you want to become a competent, confident and competitive New Grad Physio then the New Grad Physio Membership is for you.

I can accelerate your learning and in less than one year teach you the skills-sets that take many other therapists five to ten years to learn on their own, for less than the cost of most weekend courses.

When was the last time you had the perfect solution in front of you, and you stopped yourself from success?

We do this all the time. You are probably doing that right now.

You see someone else, like one of your peers, being successful, doing well, getting the right support and progressing their career much faster than everyone else – but you doubt yourself and say 'That's not me' or 'I could never do that'.

You blame external factors as an excuse for why you are not in the same position. Why? Because it's easier to take NO action than to change what you are currently doing.

It means acknowledging what you don't know and accepting you need help and support.

You are searching for a magical solution or outcome that is just going to perfectly fall into your lap.

Other New Grad Physios act and reach out for help and support as they know this is the fastest way to learn the necessary skill-sets to become a competent, confident and competitive New Grad Physio.

Which one are you going to be?

To take action visit **www.newgradphysio.com**

CHAPTER 14
New Grad Physio members in focus

To give you the insider view, here's what some of the current New Grad Physio Members are saying about how the New Grad Physio Membership has helped their own practice and helped them navigate the challenges as a New Grad Physio.

Dave Fahey – Band 5 NHS and Academy Physiotherapist at Barnsley Football Club

'Working in Academy Football I haven't been exposed to as much upper limb injury management as I would like. When the players do come in to the treatment room with upper limb injuries, I'm not confident and don't feel like I ever know enough to diagnose and treat to a good standard. I've been exposed to a lot of lower limb injuries and feel more confident with that end of things, so I have found the New Grad Physio Membership content invaluable in helping me upskill in areas and in managing injuries I lacked the experience dealing with.

'Day-to-day I'm working in ICU, in respiratory full-time, so my biggest challenge now is trying not to deskill from an MSK setting, the area where I see myself working in the long-term. I know I need to learn as much as I can, so I am ready to take my opportunity in MSK, either in the NHS or private practice, or even better in a full-time professional sports role.

'I also feel that the exposure I get to injuries that I might not normally see as part of the New Grad Physio content is filling the blanks left by university. I feel they put the 'blinkers' on us with all the teaching being geared towards working in just the NHS and therefore not as relevant to private practice and sport.

'I have worked with Andy directly recently in helping me break into a role in private practice, specifically helping me to put together a new therapy CV specific to a role in private practice. He also gave me guidance on how to avoid wasting my time, effort and money on further CPD training, instead using the New Grad Physio Membership to upskill and to guide my learning as a New Grad Physio.'

Sam Milner – Physiotherapist Coventry City Football Club

'Once I qualified, I initially found making the time and knowing how to spend my time on my continued learning difficult.

'I feel the New Grad Physio Membership, Andy and the other members in the group act to mentor me and have helped me progress. If I'm stuck with a player or presentation, I feel like I can put my questions to the group to ask for advice.

'The monthly masterclass webinars have been a huge addition to the web material as I find the short and concise content digestible and easy to learn from.

'The weekly case studies put into the Private Facebook group are helpful, particularly the atypical ones, that I may otherwise not see.

'Overall, the New Grad Physio Membership has helped me to be a more confident therapist and has helped me take my career to the next level.'

Matt Treacy – Sports Therapist Private Practice

'I joined the New Grad Physio Membership as I quickly realised upon finishing university there was so much more I needed to know. I knew I didn't have the knowledge base or know-how to apply the knowledge I had, and knew I needed guidance to help my learning progress and to direct my career.

'I have really enjoyed the New Grad Physio content and the interaction between members, particularly in the Private Facebook Group. I have also found great benefit in the different bonus modules that complement the weekly core content; they have been a great way to pool knowledge from a variety of different areas, both clinical and non-clinical.

'My main challenges working in private practice as a New Grad involved managing my caseload, being time efficient and effective with my hands-on treatments, progressing patients through a graded rehab plan and delivering a level of service to my patients that I think they deserved. The New Grad Physio Membership has helped me with all these challenges and I now feel competent and confident to deal with life as a New Grad and the challenges that present in my daily practice.'

Rhys Burton – Student Sports Therapist Leeds Beckett University
'During my student placements I have struggled to bridge the gap between making the best assessment possible and selecting the correct rehab for many different pathologies, many of which were glossed over at university.

'On a non-clinical side of things, I have found it extremely hard to create opportunities in both private practice and sport, get my foot in the door and get a job in these areas.

'Having the New Grad Physio Membership has not only given me the clinical skills I need to fill the gaps left by university, it has also given me the guidance and support I have needed to gain the opportunities to progress my career.

Having gained further experience in both professional rugby and football, I have been able to use the New Grad Physio content and skill-sets learned to provide a better level of care to the players I work with and to be adaptable with my approach to address the unique challenges each of these areas brings.'

About the New Grad Physio Mentor, Andy Barker – MSc BSc MCSP

Andy is a Consultant Physiotherapist, Private Practice Owner and The Founder and Author of *The New Grad Physio*. He currently offers consultancy to the Football Association working with England, both domestically and internationally.

Prior to this role, Andy was Head of Physiotherapy and Rehab at the Leeds Rhinos having been involved with the club for ten seasons. During this period the club enjoyed unrivalled success winning four Super League titles, two Challenge Cups and a World Club Championship.

Andy has also consulted with world level athletes from a variety of sports including boxing, professional basketball, powerlifting and extreme motorsport.

Andy graduated in Physiotherapy from the University of Bradford with a first-class honours degree which followed on from a previous Bachelor of Science degree from Leeds Metropolitan University in Sports Performance Coaching. In 2016 Andy added to this with an MSc in Sport and Exercise Biomechanics from Leeds Beckett University.

Apart from helping private practice patients and professional athletes out of pain and back to full fitness, Andy helps New Grads become competent, confident and competitive therapists by teaching them the skill-sets they need to become the next successful New Grad Physio and helping them climb the promotion ladder faster than they ever thought possible.

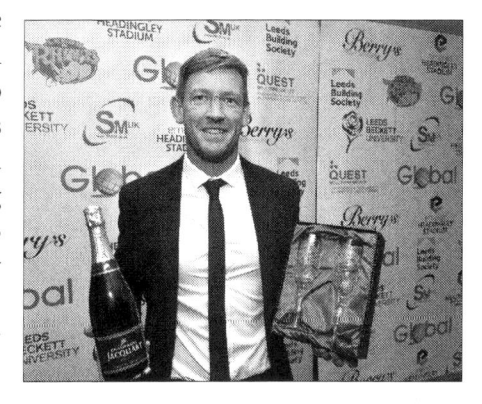

New Grad Physio bonus resources

Throughout the book I provided links to several additional resources. These resources have been created to complement the content covered in this book and further help you overcome the challenges as a New Grad and help you on your journey to becoming a competent, confident and competitive New Grad Physio.

All these resources can be accessed, completely FREE at **www.newgradphysio.com**

To find out more about the New Grad Physio Membership please visit **www.newgradphysio.com**

If you have any direct questions about your own New Grad journey and how I can help reach out to me at **andy@newgradphysio.com**

I'm also active on several social media platforms and you can find me here:

Facebook - Search 'New Grad Physio Continuing Professional Development' or use this link:
https://www.facebook.com/newgradphysio

Instagram – Search 'new grad physio' or use this link:
https://www.instagram.com/newgradphysio

LinkedIn – Search 'Andy Barker' New Grad Physio or use this link:
https://uk.linkedin.com/in/andy-barker-b9118341

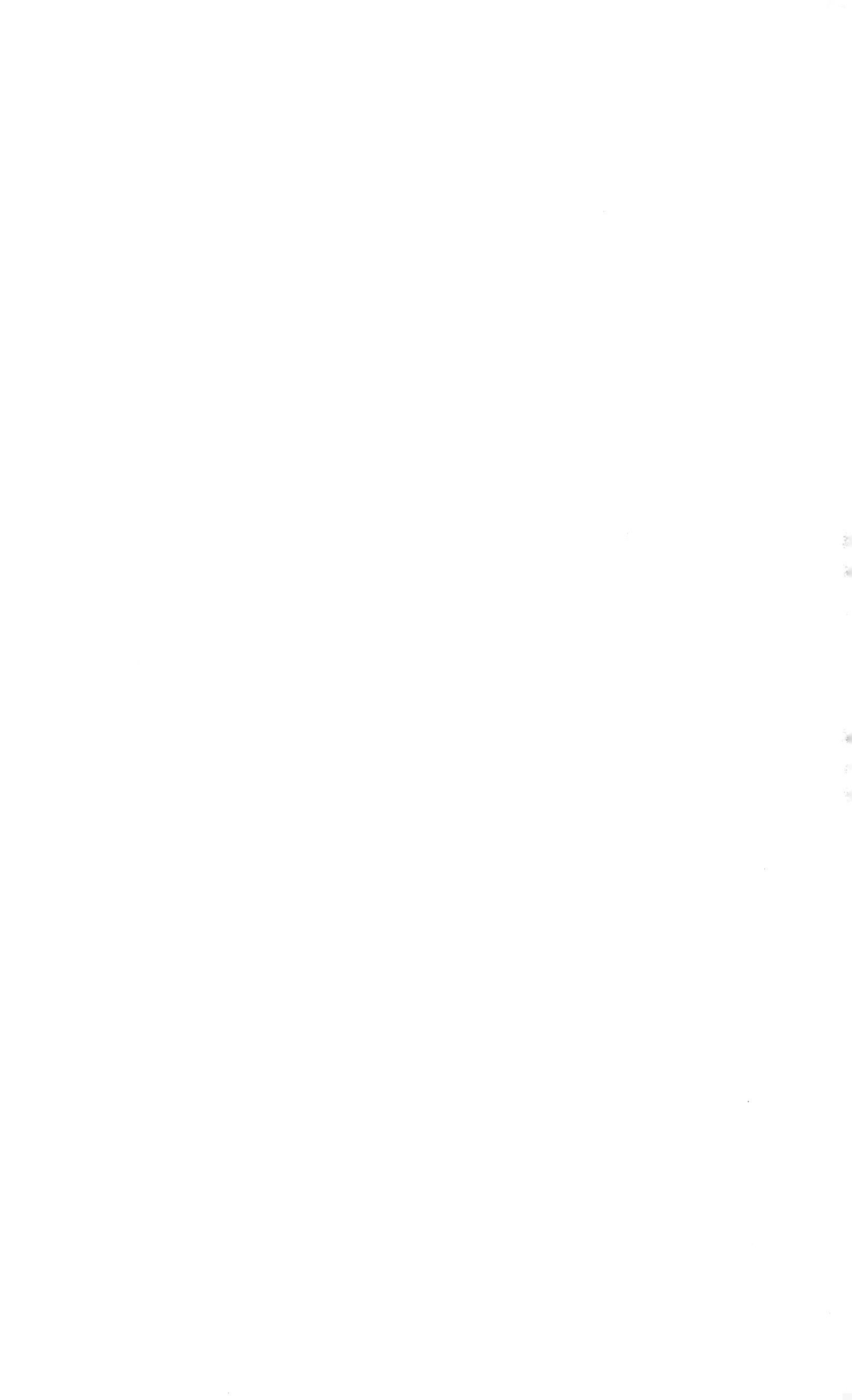

Printed in Great Britain
by Amazon